A Lighter You!

Train your Brain
to
Slim your Body

*How to Stop Dieting
and Enjoy Lasting
Weight Loss Success*

By Holly Stokes, "The Brain Trainer"
Master NLP Health Practitioner,
Certified Thought Pattern Management Practioner,
Certified NLP Life Coach, Certified Hypnotherapist

Wisdom Within Publishing

www.ALighterYouSystem.com

A Lighter You! Train Your Brain to Slim Your Body

Design by Heather Barta: www.CircleTriangleSquare.com

Photo of Holly Stokes by Kate Singh:
www.AevumImages.com

Wisdom Within Publishing
310 S. 300 W. Street
Fillmore, UT 84631

Printed in the United States of America
First printing May 2010

Disclaimer: This publication is intended to provide helpful and informative material on the subjects addressed in this book. This book and its contents are not meant to diagnose, treat, or cure illness or disease. If you are struggling with a health challenge, you are advised to continue working with your qualified health professional. Consult your medical, health, or other competent professional before adopting any of the suggestions in this book or drawing any inferences from it.

The author and publisher specifically disclaim all responsibility from any liability, loss, or risk personal or otherwise, which is incurred as a consequence, directly or indirectly, of the use and application of any of the contents of this book.

www.ALighterYouSystem.com

Table of Contents

Acknowledgments

Thank you to all the amazing clients I have had the privilege to work with over the last several years. I've learned so much from you all, and you are the inspiration behind this work.

Thank you to the wonderful professionals who took the time to review this work and offer insight, including Alison Ozgur, registered dietitian; Dianne Thomsen, registered dietitian; and Lynne Smith, family therapist, Jayne Carpenter, and others.

Thank you to all the wonderful business associates, professionals, and community members who have supported and encouraged me throughout the entire process of building my business and developing A Lighter You System.

Thank you to my colleagues who have shared their wisdom and continue to inspire me. Thank you to all my NLP teachers who are continuing to expand the field of knowledge and inspire new students.

Thank you, thank you, thank you.

Introduction

Welcome to A Lighter You System! If you are ready for a new approach, you are ready for this book. If you've lost weight only to gain it right back plus more, if you are tired of dieting and counting calories and are ready for lasting change, this book is for you.

As I look at weight loss programs, I see so many choices-countless diets, misleading media information, bad advice, and even "magic pills." Some programs are more health focused than others, but very few really help people get to the core of the problems they face.

Weight loss is a multibillion-dollar industry; yet, Americans continue to gain weight. When we think of weight loss, many of us think of eating less and exercising more; skipping meals and other forms of starvation dieting ensue. However, the body needs a certain amount of calories just to function. If we cut far below this number, it has to compensate for less energy, which it does by dumping muscle-which then lowers our metabolism. Starvation dieting can actually lower metabolism 10 to 15 percent, which is the reason why we are worse off after a diet and later gain all the weight back plus more!

Though low in calories, diet products often add lots of sugars that cause a spike in the body's blood sugar that, in turn, triggers a spike in insulin levels that can rob us of our health, leading to insulin resistance, metabolic syndrome, and diabetes.

**Diets are bad for your health!
America doesn't need another diet or magic pill;
what we really need is a mental shift!**

It's time to make peace with food and your body. Guaranteed, food and your body will be with you for the rest of your life. We don't want to avoid food, obsess about our weight, or count calories forever; we want to easily make healthy choices, nourish our body in positive ways, and let food have an easy and natural place in our lives. And, we still want to enjoy our food too!

Rather than focusing on counting calories, going hungry, feeling deprived, and yo-yo dieting, we need to address the original *causes* of weight gain. We need to change our food habits and patterns that result in extra weight. We need to address the *reasons behind* overeating, emotional eating, and the food *perceptions* that are responsible for our unhealthy food habits.

We need to change the patterns in our brain that cause the negative food habits and behaviors.

When we address these mental habits, slimming down and maintaining a healthy weight is easy! You may not believe me now, but as you read this book, you'll become more aware of your food habits and understand them. You'll also discover powerful tools and strategies to make the mental shift and quickly change the old patterns.

You may know people who don't have to worry about their weight. It's as if they can eat whatever they want-and it almost doesn't seem fair. Why do some people lose weight easily and others really struggle? If you've struggled with weight, dieted, lost weight only to gain it back again, you'll be relieved to know that there are answers, and the answers are in your brain.

The difference is in the mindset! Gung ho health nuts love to tell you "Just Do It," but it's easy for them because they already have the mindset. Many books and weight loss programs will talk about mindset, but they don't tell you how to change it.

Setting a weight loss goal usually isn't the problem. Most of us know which foods are healthy and which foods aren't. Even though we know what is healthy, we still find ourselves craving the wrong foods, eating when we are not hungry and even getting caught up in self-sabotage.

It's in following through with the plan that's difficult because it's our old habits and cravings that get in the way. Sometimes it seems the more we try to control them the worse it gets, which is why willpower alone doesn't work. These patterns can feel out of control because they are rooted in our unconscious mind and run automatically.

Just Do It Is Not Enough

The "Just Do It" theme is not enough, and as you will see in Chapter Three, willpower alone doesn't work. For lasting weight release success, we need to change our mental patterns around food and the old habits of what we think and how we feel. This book will help you understand your brain and show you how to change the old patterns that created the extra weight in the first place!

If you are ready to slim down to your healthy body naturally, have greater energy, improve your health, and feel great about you, this book is your answer! It is much more than a think-positive guide; it's a how-to guide for your brain and even for your life. As you address the underlying reasons for gaining weight, you'll feel more centered in yourself; you'll have a greater sense of well-being and even a greater ability to enjoy your life.

With this new approach-which puts you in charge of your brain-and with the right tools and right support, you'll be able to change the underlying *causes* of your habits, cravings, and even addictions. If you want *real* results and lasting change, you must engage the layers of your awareness. You must address the *root causes* of the habits and cravings, and this book will show you how.

When you are empowered with understanding your brain, knowing how it works and how to replace old habits and patterns, you'll find yourself moving forward more easily than ever before. The tools of applied psychology are expanding quickly and we no longer need to spend years struggling to create personal change. It's easier than ever to update old habits and patterns, even at the unconscious level, and take charge of your health so you can enjoy living your best life! Finally you can end the war with food and weight; you can enjoy food and let go of emotional eating, comfort eating, and stress eating and find a renewed sense of well-being with yourself and your body.

As you enjoy the healthy weight mindset and upgrade the quality of foods you are eating, you won't need to count calories and keep the numbers running in your head all day. No more diets or starving yourself either.

It's time to stop dieting! It's time to start living the lifestyle that brings you health, nutrition, fitness, and well-being. By applying these tools and principles, you'll find yourself slimming down naturally, changing your eating habits, easily maintaining your weight, increasing your energy, and feeling great about yourself.

How to Use This Book

Two parts are essential to lasting weight loss success. The first and most important part is the mental aspect-adopting the healthy weight mindset. *A Lighter You! Train your Brain to Slim your Body* is focused on this mental aspect of the equation.

The second most important part is having a solid understanding of nutrition and knowing how foods affect our bodies. Many people try to lose weight by eating less without looking at the *quality* of the foods they are choosing. It's like trying to get peak performance out of your car when you are using only bad gas. I say *eat better* not necessarily less!

To get the most out of your experience with this book, I suggest you give yourself one to two hours weekly of undisturbed time to go through the exercises. Don't read the book just once; use it as a guide to unravel your habits and cravings. Many times there are layers to the underlying reasons for carrying extra weight. Use this book over and over until you have upgraded your food choices, changed your food and health habits, and addressed the underlying patterns that have been in your way.

Each week change a mental habit and make healthy food choices. Start with small changes, it's the small steps we take every day that really add up.

It's the small steps we take every day that really add up.

Each time you go through this book, you'll find yourself adding another mental strategy, making even healthier choices, having more energy, and feeling better about yourself. You can also use the tools offered here to change patterns in other areas of your life as well. As you'll see, the areas of life and health are interconnected with mental and emotional habits. As you practice the tools offered here, you'll discover greater control in your life as you change the old patterns.

This book is written in a workbook style. You could take an hour and skim through and get the intellectual information, but the intellectual knowledge will not help you make the changes. Take your time to go through this book, *actually do the exercises*, and really use these tools to make the mental shift.

Yes, you can have the body, the health, and the life you want- and the keys to your success are in your brain! This book will give you the tools to make the mental shift, find your healthy weight mindset, and enjoy lasting weight loss success without dieting, struggling with cravings, and starving yourself. With your healthy weight mindset, slimming down and keeping your ideal healthy weight can be natural and easy.

Here are some ideas, tools, and resources that can help you get the most from this book:

Visit www.ALighterYouSystem.com where you'll find A Lighter You Membership program, extra worksheets, articles, tutorials, tele-classes, the nutrition guide, "brain training" downloads and more.

Start a support group: gather a few friends or family and start a group at your work or gym. Cover a chapter each week, going through the material in this book. Take the time to discuss what worked for you and practice the exercises with one another. This is also a great way to create a social support for you while you are making lifestyle changes.

A Lighter You! Mind Body Weight Loss Audio Course is a series of six audios designed to help you step into the healthy weight mindset. Although this book gives you the tools to begin rewiring your brain for healthy habits, the audio set takes you through a series of guided visualizations to change your perceptions of food, find motivation for exercise, upgrade the automatic programs of your deeper mind, and even change your preferences to prefer healthy choices. Listen to samples online: www.ALighterYouSystem.com

If you are using the *A Lighter You! Mind Body Weight Loss Audio Course* with this book, you'll want to listen to one CD each day for the first week, going through the whole set in the first week.

Repetition is the key to helping the brain make new habits. Repeat the audios that grab your attention first. You can listen to the audios while you are walking, stretching, doing housework, or even while falling asleep at night. As you repeat the audios, you will help your brain set up new pathways and make new habits and associations around food- and you'll find yourself slimming down to your ideal healthy you!

It's time to enjoy healthy and lasting weight loss success. With the right tools and the right support, you'll be on to your healthy weigh in no time!

Here's to your Health, Happiness, and Success!

Holly Stokes
The Brain Trainer

www.ALighterYouSystem.com

www.BrainTrainerCoach.com

Chapter One: Your Brain

Understanding Your Brain

Let's begin by taking a look at the brain and how it works. The brain is the central location for storing and processing information; it communicates to the rest of the body through the nervous system.

The body picks up information from the outside world through our five sensory channels: visual (eyes), auditory (ears), kinesthetic (touch), gustatory (taste), and olfactory (smell).

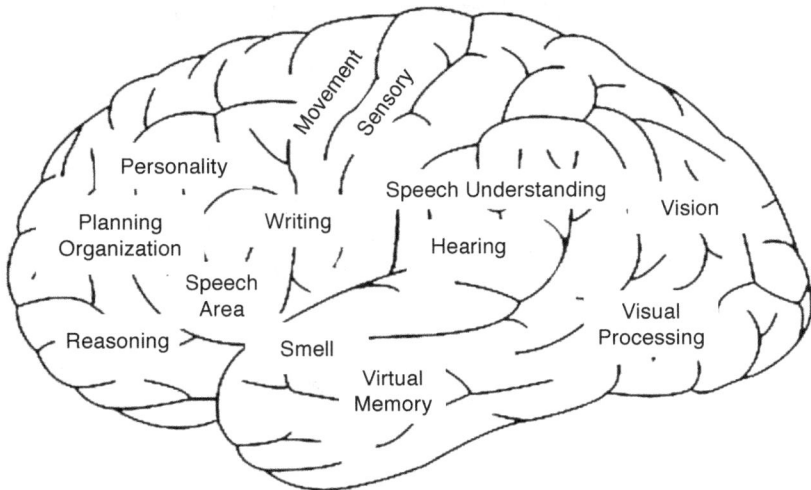

The brain uses different areas to process and store information. Incoming information from the nervous system is sorted and directed to the appropriate place in the brain for processing. Each area of the brain then stores information as memories related to that area of functioning. The visual center processes and stores visual information, the auditory information is processed through the hearing centers, body movement is processed and stored in the sensory motor area, and so on.

How the brain works is truly amazing. It was thought that the brain couldn't regenerate. But now, the brain's plasticity and ability to repair has been widely recognized. In fact, when we learn new things, our brain continues to link up neurons (nerve cells) of the brain and form new pathways.

Now, let's take a look at practical approaches to forming new pathways by engaging the different processing centers of the brain.

Neuro-Linguistic Programming and the Brain

In the 1970s, researchers Richard Bandler and Dr. John Grinder studied great communicators, therapists, and others because they were looking for the keys to human excellence and change. They wondered why some therapists have great success with clients while other therapists' clients continued to struggle. They were looking for "the difference that makes the difference."

In their research they intently observed people to identify the key strategies that offered the best results in helping people change. From their research in studying the elemental experience of making change, they laid the foundation for the study and processes of Neuro-Linguistic Programming (NLP).

Neuro refers to the neurons in the brain and nervous system, *Linguistic* refers to language, and *Programming* refers to the "programs" – or our history – that shape our perceptions. These programs act like filters that affect our daily choices and even how we see the world. The field of NLP looks at how these aspects – the brain, language, and programs – are interrelated and how they make up our experience.

NLP has developed into a field of study with hundreds of processes to help people create change. In working with NLP for several years, I have found these tools extremely effective both with clients and for myself. With my clients, NLP has boosted the effectiveness of hypnosis, increased the speed of integrating deep-level change, and sped up the cycle of the whole change process. NLP is so effective because the tools and strategies engage the different processing centers of the brain, creating a better "reminder" system for the change we want to create:

Visualization: Engages the visual part of the brain.

Speaking and Hearing: Engages the language and speech centers of the brain.

Walking and Moving: Engages the sensory and motor centers of the brain.

Symbols and Imagery: Engages the brain's creative centers and speaks to the unconscious mind.

By engaging more of the brain's processing centers – visualization, speaking and hearing, walking and moving, and symbols and imagery – we can engage more of our brain and our body's nervous system in making the new change.

Many of the tools I present in this book come from the field of NLP. NLP allows us to take control of how the brain is working, set up new habits quickly, and change old patterns. We can even tap into patterns that are deeply ingrained in our unconscious mind and update them quickly and effectively.

The founding principles of NLP help us to better understand human experience. The field continues to grow; there are now hundreds of processes that can help rewire the brain for anything from changing habits to changing trauma responses and fears, to updating old beliefs or programs, to improving motivation and performance in any area of life.

It's amazing the results when you understand how your brain works and how to put it to work for you. Finally, with what we know now about the brain and how it works, it's easier than ever to make the change you desire.

Your Unconscious Mind

Another aspect to how our mind operates is more elusive but very important in how it affects our daily choices and motivations.

Have you ever experienced self-sabotage? You may have felt, "It's as if a part of me wants to and a part of me doesn't," or it's as if the devil is on one shoulder and an angel is on the other and you find yourself caught between the two. You may even have argued with yourself over bad food choices, dieting, or exercise, or you may have set a goal not to eat sweets but then didn't catch yourself until after you finished the cookie.

If we really want to end the battle with food, weight, and our bodies, we simply must address this elusive yet powerful aspect of how we operate.

Consciously, you may have decided that you are *100 percent this time going to lose weight.* A few days roll by and you lose motivation, find excuses, or rationalize the extra helpings or sweets. Even though consciously you set a goal and know what you want, if your deeper mind is not aligned with your conscious goal, but has a different agenda, you will continue to struggle.

You may have found that you can swear off sugar for a few days or a week, but then the compulsion to eat it comes back even stronger. Fighting against what the unconscious mind wants can create a backlash, which is why denying and depriving ourselves just doesn't work. In fact, this cycle of discipline and deprivation is a recipe for binge eating-when the compulsion builds until it is out of control. There is now a better and more effective way to update these old programs or desires of the unconscious mind.

By using the language of the unconscious mind and working with your deeper awareness, you can engage your deeper mind to work *for* you rather than against you. So, let's take a look at the layers of the mind and how they influence our lives and choices.

From the world of psychology, Sigmund Freud popularized the understanding of the layers of the mind. I like to use the image of an iceberg to explain these layers.

Think of an iceberg. About 10 percent of the iceberg is the portion we see above water, which is like our conscious mind. Our **conscious** mind is great for planning and setting goals, for logic and reasoning. This is our day-to-day awareness.

Now, just below the surface is the **subconscious** mind. Here we keep information that is easy to retrieve, information that we repeat often or that is recent. For example, remembering your phone number or address falls into this category; this information is easy to remember because we review it often.

Now, think of your fifth birthday. How much do you remember? You probably don't remember much unless you have photos to remind you. Just because you don't consciously remember something, however, doesn't mean it didn't happen. All memories, experiences, and events are stored in the **unconscious** mind.

For efficiency, our brain stacks memories one on top of the other, with the older memories at the bottom of the pile. The more recent events and the more often-reviewed events are higher up on the pile and therefore easier to remember. We don't need to remember the older memories daily; we need just the information we use often or recently.

Now, think of children. During the first years of life their brains are in explosive growth. They are learning a new language, learning to coordinate a little body, discovering how the world operates, learning social cues, and more. Their brains are like sponges soaking up everything in their environment. In the early years the brain is learning, creating associations and meanings by making neural connections. When we learn, the brain links up neurons and creates neural pathways that lay the foundation for how we see the world. These pathways are responsible for the habits and patterns in the brain.

During our formative years, what we learn about ourselves and how life works affects how we see the world. The events of our past shape our perception and, much like a pair of glasses, create a filter of how we see the world. Our entire history is stored in our deeper mind along with all the meanings we've attached to that history. And it's our *history* that affects the daily choices we make even if we are not consciously aware of those underlying reasons.

So for any given event, our unconscious mind reviews our history and sums up the positive and negative, and then we get a feeling about it. We have feelings associated with different foods, with exercise, the refrigerator, our relationships, and more. These feelings translate into our motivations and our choices.

If you've struggled with the same goal or challenge over and over, it's because a deeper part of your mind doesn't want the change. When these automatic programs are working against our conscious goals, what we experience is self-sabotage. The unconscious mind runs many automatic programs for us as habits. Many are helpful, but sometimes they are outdated, operating from old rules and reasons based on our history and experiences.

I was teaching a weight loss and healthy lifestyle class and it was week four. As my students filed in, I started class with the question, "So what are you doing for exercise?" I got blank stares. "It's week four now, you know you are supposed to be adding in exercise." More silence.

Suddenly, one of the ladies blurted out, "If we liked to exercise we wouldn't be here!"

My NLP ears perked up and I asked, "Okay, so when you think of exercise what comes to mind?"

The ladies took turns: "Sweaty!" "Stinky!" "Hard!" "Yuck!"

Because of their history with exercise, these ladies had negative feelings attached to the concept of exercise. Our unconscious mind scans through the history, both positive and negative, and sums it up with a feeling. If we have negative feelings connected to an activity, we are less motivated to do it.

Our unconscious mind usually speaks to us through feelings. It's also active when we are sleeping and often uses symbolism, imagery, and metaphor while we sleep. We can update the automatic programs our unconscious mind operates by speaking in its own language: using images, pictures, symbols, and feelings more than words and logic. This is why guided visualizations work so well: we are speaking to our unconscious mind using its own language.

Especially meaningful to our unconscious mind is imagery and metaphor. Milton Erickson (1901-1980), a renowned hypnotherapist, was famous for telling stories that resolved a person's problem. By recognizing the unconscious mind's ability to learn and find new solutions, he often simply told his clients stories that the mind could learn from and apply, sometimes instantly changing the problem.

If you want to engage your unconscious mind to work for you rather than against you, you must speak its language and give it clear directions. In fact, our unconscious mind is always listening, but we may not be aware of the directions we are giving it. As you travel through this book, you'll find better ways to update your unconscious mind so that you can set it up to work *for* you rather than against you.

Creating alignment within ourselves is essential to creating effective and lasting change. If we want to truly stop struggling, we must work with our deeper awareness rather than fight against our unconscious programs. When we've aligned the part of us that doesn't want to move forward with our conscious goals, making the change and keeping it becomes so much easier. It seems as if it almost happens overnight!

The Power of Language

Pay attention to your words and self-talk because your unconscious mind is always listening. It scans all the meanings around our words and uses pictures to interpret our language. Those mental images speak even more directly to our unconscious mind than our words do. As you pay attention to your language, you'll engage your unconscious to work for you.

Whatever we focus on will grow. If you are focusing on the problem-guess what? The *problem gets bigger,* if only in your mind!

When we talk about a weight loss goal, we often say, "I want to lose 20 pounds." We understand the meaning consciously, but that deeper part of our mind-the unconscious-is also listening when we speak, and it sums up all our history and meanings of the words we use.

Try this: Say the phrase "I want to lose 20 pounds" and pay attention to how you feel when you say it. What does that phrase draw to your attention? You'll probably notice the feeling of being fat or the extra 20 pounds that you *don't want*.

Now, think of the common phrase "weight loss." When you say this phrase, what do you think of? Another meaning of the word *weight* is *wait* as in stop, and the word *loss* is usually connected with sadness.

Do you feel great about things you've lost? After we've lost something, we often spend a lot of time and energy trying to find it again. Have you ever lost your weight only to find it again? In a sense, even the phrase "weight loss" could be getting in your *weigh* because your unconscious is hearing *wait* -be sad and go find what you lost.

If you say, "I don't want to be heavy anymore," what pictures come to your mind? That's right, being heavy. Consciously we understand the word *don't*, but it doesn't translate into mental pictures, and our unconscious mind uses mental pictures to interpret our words.

I'm going to ask you not to do something; see how well you can follow directions. Don't think of a yellow butterfly because as you do, it will flap its wings, turn blue, and fly out of the room.

What did your mind do? It pictured the butterfly. Remember: In order to understand the words you use, your mind uses mental pictures. Even though you consciously understand *don't*, that word doesn't translate into mental pictures, and those pictures are speaking directly to your unconscious mind.

Our unconscious mind is always listening to what we are telling it, but the language of the unconscious mind operates in pictures, images, symbols, and feelings more than in words. If we want our unconscious mind to work with us, we need to give it clear directions of what we want in its own language. By focusing on what you want and using *language that focuses* on what you want rather than on what you *don't* want, you give your unconscious mind positive directions.

**Focus on what you want
rather than on what you don't want.**

Notice what you picture in your mind and how you feel when you say, "I desire to be my ideal healthy weight."

Keep your mind focused on what you *do want:* Your Ideal Healthy Weight.

What is the ideal healthy weight you want to be? Pick your number:

Use positive language to help your mind and body embrace this image of you. Using words that offer you positive images and feelings will better support you in *becoming* your ideal body image. Even better, use this phrase: "I *am becoming* my ideal healthy self."

Pay attention to the words you use. Instead of saying "I am losing weight," say, "I am letting go of extra weight" or "I am releasing fat" (that's right; you don't have to *hold onto it* anymore). The healthy you is already within you!

Here are some better ways to phrase your "weight loss" goal:

I am letting go of the extra weight.

I am becoming my ideal healthy self.

I am becoming my ideal size.

I am embracing my ideal body shape.

I am embodying my healthy weight number:

Notice how these phrases draw your attention and focus to being the body you want. Notice how you feel when you say the phrases; even the words you choose can motivate and inspire you!

As you begin to notice and change your language, you can shift your perceptions and find more motivation as you affect the action, thought, and feeling cycle.

The Action, Thought, and Feeling Cycle

When we think of goals, we are often very focused on action, but whether we follow through or not requires more than action. In fact, if we focus on just the action piece of the equation, we are missing most of the battle.

Most of us know that we can release weight by eating more fruits and vegetables and making healthier choices. But what gets in our way are the old habits, cravings, and even self-sabotage.

Setting a goal for weight release is the easy part; it's following through that is difficult. What keeps us from staying on track with a goal? It's almost as if a part of us wants to change and a part of us doesn't, and then we struggle between these two parts.

If we are to end the struggle, the yo-yo dieting, and release the weight naturally, we need to understand that what we think, feel, and do are all interconnected. If we want to experience lasting change, we need to change the quality of the thoughts and feelings from which we operate.

Our actions, thoughts and feelings are all interconnected. If we want to change our actions, we need to change the quality of our thoughts and feelings.

What we think and feel daily are mental habits. These habits are wired into our brain, as we'll see in more detail in the next chapter. Many times we don't even notice that these thought and feeling habits are running through our mind because they happen so quickly.

If we focus just on changing behavior, we will continue to struggle. For lasting results, we simply must address these mental patterns – the thinking and feeling habits – and replace them with new patterns. When we are thinking better and feeling better, we do better.

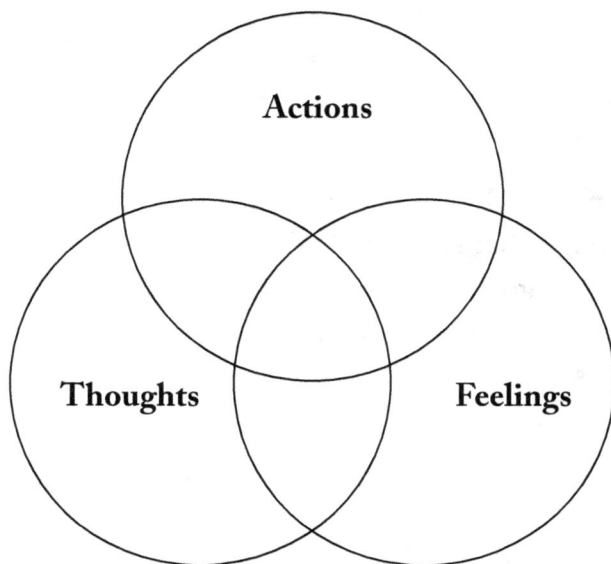

As a coach, I often help clients become clear about what they want and then set a goal. Setting a goal is what we do with our conscious, action-planning mind. Setting a goal is great, but it's only part of the picture. When we pick a goal but ignore the underlying thoughts and feelings that drive us, we set ourselves up for failure.

What gets in our way of following through are *feelings*, such as lack of motivation and even cravings and self-sabotage. These kinds of feelings are not from our conscious, action-planning mind; they are generated from our deeper awareness, even from our unconscious mind. When we think about something we want to do, our deeper mind scans through our history, both the good and the bad, and sums it up for us with a feeling.

Motivation is a key to our success – and motivation is a feeling! But how do we get motivated? How do we tap into our deeper self and engage our inner drive?

If you affect one component of the action-thought-feeling cycle, it affects the other components as well. This is how we get stuck in a downward spiral: If I feel down about myself and reach for comfort foods and then berate myself for eating it saying, "I'm not disciplined." Then, from the self criticism and guilt, I feel worse and so reach for more comfort foods, which causes me to gain weight, feel bad about myself and so I reach for more comfort food… and the cycle continues.

Or you can use the same principle of affecting the action-thought-feeling cycle to engage an upward spiral. If I give myself positive encouragement, I feel good about myself. As I feel good about myself, I have more energy, as I have more energy, I feel more motivated to follow through on my goals. As I feel motivated, I take action, as I take action I feel better about myself and so on and so on.

As you go through this book, you'll notice how your thoughts, feelings, and actions interact and affect your choices and motivation.

The Problems with Setting Goals

When we think of weight loss, often we start with a weight loss goal. We may even have a number in mind and say, "I want to lose 20 pounds." We might even feel motivated and make the commitment. If we are really detailed, we may even make it a **SMARTER** goal (Specific, Measurable, Achievable, Realistic, on a Timeline, Evaluate, and Review). But setting a goal doesn't mean we'll actually follow through with it.

Before you get going, you need to be aware that there is a problem with setting goals. Don't get me wrong; goal setting is important, but often we sabotage ourselves even before we start. To better understand our hang-ups with goals, let's take a look at the Goal-Setting Cycle.

First, we have the thought that we want something different in our lives. I want to be healthier, slimmer, or more fit. We see where we are now versus where we'd like to be, and where we'd like to be becomes the goal. If we are really detailed, we might get specific and write down how we will accomplish the goal and by when. If we are really really detailed, we might even break it down into steps we will take every day.

Then, a few days roll by and maybe we do pretty well, but after a few more days we procrastinate, we're just not feeling motivated. We find we don't have the time, maybe we forget; maybe other things take priority-until we've totally fallen off the wagon.

But that's not the end of the Goal-Setting Cycle! We then berate ourselves for not staying on track, maybe even call ourselves names, saying "I'm just lazy" or "I'm not disciplined enough," and we then feel bad about not following through. Finally, we tuck the goal into the graveyard along with all those other goals that have gone before.

Then, the next time we decide to set a goal, we get visitations from the ghosts of goals past. "Remember what happened last time," echoes in our head, or "you're just lazy and undisciplined; what makes you think it will work this time?" Because of the history of the goals undone and the negative feelings attached, we might even give up before we start.

When you think of goals, what comes to your mind? Quite possibly, it's all the goals sleeping in the graveyard and the ghosts of goals past.

Problem #1: We have history attached to our goals. And more likely than not, that history has negative associations with it so we never really start with a clean slate. Calling it a healthy weight *plan* rather than a goal can take the pressure off, with less emphasis on success and failure. Plans have more wiggle room; plans can adjust and change.

While you are defining your plan, recognize that this time it will be different. Recognize what you are doing differently now that will make a difference for you. You have new resources, new ideas, and better ways of moving forward – especially with the material in this book.

Problem #2: We have rigid ideas of success and failure attached to our goals. If we do not reach the goal 100 percent by the timeline, it becomes a failure even though we may have made progress.

With such a history of goals and failures in the graveyard, the process of setting a goal may seem daunting, and bring up feelings of guilt and failure. We may feel the wind go out of our sails even before we get started. It's no wonder why most people don't set goals, even setting a goal can get in our way.

Let's take a moment now to rethink *failure*. If you give a child a bicycle, how many chances does he get to learn to ride? He gets as many as it takes.

And if he falls off the bike, would you say he failed?

Of course not. Even though the child may fall off, he is still learning. The mind and body are taking note of the adjustments that need to be made. The brain is making calculations about balance and coordination, and the next time the child saddles the bike, it becomes easier and he is more successful. The child gets as many chances as it takes to learn to ride the bicycle.

So, really, in the picture of learning and growing there is no failure; there is only learning and results. If you don't like your results, it's simply time to make some changes and adjustments.

Rather than focusing on what isn't working, focus on what is working. As you notice what's working, you can do more of what's working so you can get the results you want. Maybe you have learned a lot about weight release and what doesn't work for you, and with all the *learning* you've been doing, it will be so much easier to move forward in a new way!

Make these agreements with yourself now:

Failure doesn't exist; there is only learning and results.

I choose to recognize my learning so I can get better results.

I agree to notice what is working for me so I can do more of what's working for me.

Problem #3: We hold our happiness hostage with our goals. We identify where we are, we know where we want to be, and the distance from here to there becomes the goal. Then we put our happiness off into the land of someday.

I will be happy someday . . .

• When I have lost 20 pounds, then I will feel good about myself.

• When I become a size 9 or 10, then I can appreciate my body.

• When I lose the weight, then I will enjoy life more.

The secret is this: It's not really just about accomplishing the goal; it's also about what *we think the goal will get for us.* What we really want is the *higher feeling* we think the goal will bring to our lives.

The higher feeling is actually the key to our motivation. If we think we can have the feeling only when we've achieved the goal, it's like we're holding a carrot in front of ourselves and never getting the reward. We'll probably continue to feel unsatisfied, struggle with motivation, and feel unfulfilled.

Think of a goal you chose that you thought would bring you happiness. As you look back now, you may notice that even after you achieved the goal your mind was already onto the next thing. Perhaps you picked another goal and pushed your happiness farther back into the land of someday without even realizing it.

If we are not paying attention to the *higher purpose* of our goal or plan, we will continue to sabotage our happiness, hold ourselves hostage, and feel frustrated with ourselves. If we are not paying attention to what we think our plan will bring us, we could be sabotaging our efforts without knowing it.

The real secret behind the plan is this:
It's not just about the goal or plan - it's really about
the higher feeling we think our plan will bring us.

I call this higher feeling the Plan's Higher Purpose. Each plan has two parts: the defined actions for achieving the plan, and the higher feeling you think achieving the plan will bring you, the Plan's Higher Purpose.

Define Your Higher Purpose

Ask the Magic Question: What will this get for me? As you answer this question, ask it again. Keep asking and answering this question until you follow the answers to your plan's higher purpose. It will show up as a feeling. You will find that the higher purpose of your plan is really about a feeling or a sense of something.

Ask yourself: If my plan is to weigh 150 pounds, what will that get for me?

Answer: If I were to weigh 150 pounds, my clothes will fit better.

Ask yourself: What will my clothes fitting better get for me?

Answer: I will feel more comfortable in my body.

Ask yourself: What will that get for me?

Answer: I will be able to move more and have more *freedom*.

Ask yourself: What will that get for me?

Answer: I can feel good about myself and enjoy life more.

From this example, we can see that the weight loss plan represents *feeling good about myself and enjoying life more*, not just weighing 150 pounds.

Letting go of the extra weight is really about the higher feeling you think weight loss will bring you.

The Real Secret Behind Our Plans

Here is the secret behind the plan's higher feeling: We don't have to wait until we've achieved the plan to connect with this feeling. We can have this feeling now! We don't have to wait until we've done x, y, or z to have this feeling.

Think of the higher feeling of your plan. Now, think of the activities that help you connect with that feeling. Enjoying life more can be as simple as a bubble bath; peace of mind can be a 15-minute walk during lunch break; appreciating yourself can be as easy as creating a list of what you like about yourself and reviewing it regularly. Enjoying life more can be making time in your life for the things you really love to do.

What we really want is the *higher feeling* we think the plan will bring us. If we aren't paying attention to our higher purpose, however, it is like spinning on a hamster wheel – setting a goal, falling off the wagon, beating ourselves up, and repeating the old cycle of "failing" until we are downtrodden and don't want to try again. We don't allow ourselves the carrot, the higher feeling because we haven't completed the goal. So, we feel unsatisfied, defeated, and even hopeless about repeating a goal.

Don't weight (yes, pun intended) to lose the pounds so you can feel good about yourself, indulge in the positive feeling that you are searching for and enjoy the higher benefit now!

We can access positive feelings even as quickly as we think about them.

What we really need is a paradigm shift! We hold ourselves hostage with our goals, thinking we can't feel good about ourselves, or feel accomplished, or have the carrot at the end of the stick until we've achieved the goal. No wonder we feel frustrated!

How many times have you set a goal and found you didn't fulfill the goal 100 percent? It left you hanging, you probably didn't feel satisfied, and you didn't get what you really wanted – *which was really a feeling!*

The real truth is, the carrot is the fuel for our motivation! As we feel better, we think better and as we do better. If you want to release the weight, you need to truly nourish yourself at all levels. So, don't wait to reach your ideal size to get what you *really* want – *the higher feeling.* Connect with those positive feelings in your life now. You'll enjoy the whole journey so much more!

**The motivation we are looking for
comes from connecting with our higher feeling
even before we've achieved the goal.**

My Plan

Take a few moments to think about your plan. Here is a worksheet for you to use in helping you clarify your plan, identify your higher purpose, and start making room for the higher purpose in your life.

What is your Plan? _____

_____

What will that get for me? _____

_____

What will that get for me? _____

_____

What will that get for me? _____

_____

The higher feeling (or higher purpose) of releasing weight is:

_____

_____

Part of the key to success is to create the higher feeling for yourself now. Think of the higher feeling. What simple ways can you connect with it now in your life? Take a moment to brainstorm.

Empowering yourself with the positive feelings of your higher benefit then becomes part of your focus for success. From the list above, what can you begin introducing in your life now to bring that positive feeling? These activities can be as simple as taking just 5 minutes. Brainstorm, then pick your top three.

Turn your higher feeling into a positive phrase to remind yourself to connect with that higher feeling. Post your phrases in places you will see regularly – the door as you leave your house for the day, the refrigerator, the mirror in the bathroom:

I can feel good about myself today.

I can enjoy life more.

I can relax and appreciate myself.

Part of your focus in being successful is to reward yourself. Rather than holding the carrot in front of you, give yourself what you *really* want along the way. These positive feelings will help inspire and motivate you. Using the word *can* in these phrases opens your mind to the possibility of it, making the feelings more reachable.

Now, let's put it all together. With your new formula for achievement and success, you can begin to focus your attention on what you want in a positive way and feel great about the process.

New Formula for Achievement and Success

Step 1: Turn Your Goal into a Plan: Use positive language. Rather than saying, "I want to lose 20 pounds," say, "I am becoming my ideal healthy body."

Plans change; they have flexibility and wiggle room, and we don't have the same ideas of success and failure attached as we do with having a goal. It's easier to have a plan than a goal.

Step 2: Identify Your Plan's Higher Purpose: Remember, we are not calling it a goal anymore. What is it the plan will bring you? If you ask the magic question a few times, you will find that the higher purpose is really a feeling. From the higher purpose exercise you finished, identify the higher feeling you are looking for from your plan.

Your Plan: _____

Plan's Higher Purpose (the feeling): _____

_____

Step 3: Make Your Plan SMARTER: (Specific, Measurable, Achievable, Realistic, on a Timeline, Evaluate, and Review):

Keep it Specific (and simple): Pick only two or three actions you will take each week that will bring you closer to your desired outcome. What will you do daily and weekly? What times will you set aside for these actions? There is magic in the small actions that we do every day – it's these small steps that really add up.

The best-laid plans are those we do every day. We are creatures of habit, and when you create new habits during your day, you will find it easier and easier to follow through until they become part of your lifestyle.

Food and Nourishment Plans: Most of us know we'd be healthier by eating more fresh fruits and vegetables. Here are some ideas for just that focus: include one fruit each day and eat two vegetables for dinner, take lunch with you to work instead of eating out, keep fresh fruits visually available and reach for them in place of sweets. If you need more ideas and more nutrition information, visit the website for the nutrition guide: www.ALighterYouSystem.com

Fitness Plans: When people think of losing weight, often they begin heroic fitness efforts, only to find they burn out in a few days or weeks. Giant efforts in exercise and starvation just leave us exhausted and frustrated and likely to give up. Your fitness plans shouldn't focus on exhaustive hours at the gym, especially in the beginning. In fact, if you aren't used to exercising, start with just 10 minutes. Keep it reasonable and add more activities and time as you enjoy it more and increase your endurance.

Keep it Fun! Identify the activities you enjoy and add them into your day and week. Invite your friends or family to enjoy fitness time with you. Fitness goals can include a 10-15 minute walk during your lunch break, playing with your kids at the park, family game night, bike riding, hiking, swimming – anything that gets you moving. If you pick activities you love and enjoy doing, you will stick with them, decrease your stress, and *enjoy life more.* What fitness activities do you love and enjoy? It's not good just for your body, it's good for your mental health and well-being.

Measurable: The total number of pounds you want to let go of: ____

Achievable and Realistic: Healthy weight reduction is really about 1-2 pounds per week, so take your Measurable number of pounds (above) and divide by 2. That number is your timeline, the total number of weeks you can expect to achieve your healthy weight. Keep your focus long term; creating healthy change is all about the healthy habits that will continue to support you through the rest of your life and is not just another diet. For lasting success, you will be creating a lifestyle that is balanced and that works for you.

Your Timeline: Total number of pounds divided by 2 = total weeks: _____

Evaluate and Review: Set aside time to evaluate your progress – what's worked for you and what hasn't worked as well. Part of your plan can be to set aside one hour a week to do the exercises in this book as you find the thought and feeling patterns you'd like to change.

Working with a support group, coach, or personal trainer, or checking in with a friend or partner can help you stay on track and motivated. Make sure the person you check in with is someone who believes in you. By checking in with someone who holds you accountable, you will be more focused in following through, which can add momentum to your program, especially in the beginning while you are making healthy changes.

I recommend a weekly review. Look at what you did that worked and what didn't work. What got in your way of your success? Perhaps you found yourself giving in to a craving, eating for comfort or emotional reasons. As you identify what patterns are getting in your way, you can use the tools in this book to set you up for more success each week.

If you aren't following through, it simply means you need to make some adjustments. What can you change, adjust, or shift to set you up for more success the next week?

Rewards: Remember to reward your successes! Give yourself rewards and *make sure your rewards fit your higher purpose.* For example, if my higher purpose in releasing fat is to feel healthier and feel good about myself, rewarding with a sundae is not the best fit. A better reward may be a massage, buying clothes that help me feel attractive and confident, or taking the time for creative activities that really nourish me and help me connect with feeling good about myself and my body.

What are some ways you can reward yourself that help you connect with your plan's higher purpose?

Keep your higher benefit in mind and use the following table to define your milestones of success and how you will celebrate your success along the way. Make sure your rewards match your higher purpose! Choose celebrations that further this "sense of something" for you.

Milestones	Celebrations	Target Date	Date Achieved
Release 10 lbs.			
Next 10 lbs.			
Next 10 lbs.			
Next 10 lbs.			

Step 4: Put the Plan in Your Planner: If it's not written down, it's not going to happen. By setting aside the time in your planner, you're more likely to remember and follow through. Treat your times as appointments with yourself. If something comes up, reschedule it just like you would a regular appointment.

When my clients say, "I will exercise three times this week," I always ask, "What days will work best for you? What times of day will fit your schedule best?" Often, as they think about it, they have to change their plans to fit their schedules.

Make sure your action steps will work for you and your life. Where do these actions best fit your life? Map it out and put it in your planner. Your steps may look like this:

Sun.	Mon.	Tues.	Wed.	Thurs.	Fri.	Sat.
5-6 Review with Coach	11:30-12 walking		11:30-12 walking		11:30-12 walking	9-10 Study group

Create a checklist of your activities for the week so you can track your progress (pick 2-3 activities per week at most). Place it somewhere you will see it often; on the refrigerator is a great place. Your weekly chart can be as simple as this:

Activity	Sun	Mon	Tue	Wed	Thu	Fri	Sat
Eat one fresh fruit daily							
Bring lunch to work							
Exercise 15 min. 3 times per week							

Here is a sample plan:

The Plan: Release 20 pounds – weigh 150 pounds

The Higher Purpose: Feel good about myself, enjoy life more.

What I will do to achieve this: I will eat better and incorporate movement and fitness into my week.

Simple and Specific:

I will eat better: I will bring my lunch to work rather than eating at fast food places; I will eat at least one fresh fruit a day and at least two vegetables with dinner.

I will incorporate movement: I will walk for 15 minutes during my lunch break and I will take the time for more exercise during the weekends.

Measurable: Total number of pounds to release: 20

Achievable and Realistic Timeline: 10 weeks

Evaluate and Review: Weekly, Sundays 5-6 pm.

Reward Successes: I will take a half-day for myself to relax and enjoy life; I'll go for a walk along the river.

My Healthy Life Plan Worksheet

My Weight Plan: (State it in the positive):

My Plan's Higher Purpose: (What is the higher feeling you think weight loss will bring you, and how can you have that feeling in your life now?)

My Simple and Specific Plane: What activities will you do daily and weekly? Pick just 2-3 (activities each week.)

Measurable:
Total number of pounds to release: _____

Achievable and Realistic Timeline:
Total number of lbs divided by 2 = number of weeks I can expect: _____

Evaluation and Review:

When and Where?

With whom?

What will you do in your review?

Milestones	Reward Success	Target Date	Date Achieved
Release 10lbs.			
Next 10lbs.			
Next 10lbs.			
Next 10lbs.			

Cue-ing Your Brain into Your Plan

Now that you've created your plan, you can engage your brain to help you stay on track. Often when we choose a goal, we see it way off in the future in the land of someday. Many times when we choose a goal, we have a concept about the end result, but the end result itself isn't clearly defined and is shrouded in mystery.

By taking the time to imagine your plan *achieved* as if you have it now, you are experiencing the end result in a way that makes your plan more real, more tangible, and more achievable. You are also telling your deeper mind to take on this better image of you and try on your positive future.

We can give the brain clear directions about what we want to achieve by engaging its different processing centers. As we do, we are adding to those processing centers new visual, auditory, and kinesthetic information – essentially updating the brain.

Using imagination is also a way to engage your unconscious mind to update with your conscious desires. It's a great way to connect with what you want because those mental pictures are telling your unconscious mind what you want it to do.

Take a moment now to sit, relax, and imagine you already are the ideal healthy you. Imagine seeing your ideal healthy body in the mirror. Hear yourself saying positive encouragement, and notice how your body feels as the ideal healthy you. Imagine what it is like being you in your ideal healthy body.

Visual: What do you see?

Auditory: What do you hear?

Kinesthetic: What do you feel?

As you connect with your positive picture of yourself, it will feel more real to you, more reachable and achievable rather than way off somewhere in the land of someday. As you imagine yourself having achieved your results, you are telling your unconscious mind what you want it to do for you.

Stepping into Your Ideal Healthy Weight

Now that you have imagined yourself in your healthy body, write your story from the perspective of having achieved lasting success. Looking back from that place in the future to where you are now, offer yourself some positive advice for the process.

What positive and encouraging advice would you give yourself?

What benefits have you found through your weight release and healthy body journey?

Bring that awareness of your future self all the way back to now, and even as you do, your unconscious mind can create the roadmap for moving forward as your ideal healthy self. As you imagine the experience of your future self, it becomes more real and achievable for you. Imagination also tells your unconscious mind in pictures where you want it to take you!

Brain Reminders

Sometimes creating a change is as simple as remembering to do it. You can create reminders for your brain that are focused on the results you want to achieve. Place these reminders where you will see them often. Create visual reminders (as in the picture below), auditory reminders (as in word cues), and kinesthetic reminders (as in touch and feeling cues).

Visual Cues: Picturing Yourself as the Ideal Healthy You*

To help your mind identify with your healthy ideal weight, find a picture of what you want your body to look like. You can use magazine photos, but choose realistic pictures. (Caution: Be aware that the photos of models in magazines have been airbrushed; they don't really look like that.) Even better is to use a photo of you from an earlier time.

Then take a current photo of just your face, cut it out, and paste it on your "after" body. Or, use a separate paper and post your "after" self in places where you will see it – the refrigerator or a mirror. When you see it, you will be reminded of the healthy you that you are becoming!

*"Step Into the Healthy You," Disc #1 of A Lighter You! Mind Body Weight Loss Audio Course, focuses on helping your mind identify with the image of the lighter, healthier you. Use the visualization to help your mind cue into the image of your ideal body. More worksheets and planning tools are available at www.ALighterYouSystem.com.

Remember that our unconscious mind speaks in pictures, images, and symbols more than in words. By using some visual cues, you are engaging your deeper mind to help you on the journey.

Auditory Cues

Auditory cues can be as simple as posting positive words and reminders in places you see often. I like posting on mirrors, the refrigerator, or even on my computer. Repeating your positive phrases out loud will then store them in your speech and hearing centers.

I can be a healthy size and weight.

I am becoming my ideal healthy self.

I am slimming into my lighter self.

Kinesthetic Cues

Kinesthetic cues relate to what you can touch and feel; they can tie into the positive messages you post. When you say these phrases, allow yourself to connect with the positive feelings. Here are some good examples of kinesthetic cues.

I *feel good* about myself as I am releasing weight.

I *appreciate* my body and all that it does for me.

My *body feels good* in my clothes.

I *enjoy* being me.

Positive Agreements

Here are some agreements to help you create a solid foundation for being successful in releasing weight. Take a moment to read through them, check off the ones you are willing to do, and circle the ones when you notice resistance. The following chapters will show you how to release resistance and break free of old patterns.

I am ready and willing to try new things.

I am ready to commit to my own health and well-being.

I am ready to create a new relationship with myself and my body.

I realize my health is a reflection of how well I care for myself.

I give myself permission to take care of me, to make the time for planning, preparation, and self-reflection throughout the week.

I agree to pay attention to my body and what is right for me.

I agree to stop blaming myself and others, and I agree to take full responsibility for all my results.

I agree to be patient with my results; although others may get faster results, I appreciate that my body has its own wisdom and timing for releasing the extra weight.

I agree to be persistent in my efforts and recognize that so-called mistakes are part of the learning process.

I agree to be aware of my own emotional states, habits, and patterns so I can change them.

I agree to let go of the things (thoughts and feelings) that are no longer working for me.

Chapter Two:
Keys to Changing Habits

What Is a Habit?

Our brain creates habits for efficiency. Anything we repeat over time becomes a habit. This is useful in many ways: we no longer need to repeatedly learn to tie our shoes or drive a car; we do it on autopilot.

We also have habits that are not so useful. Changing a habit used to be hard to do, but not anymore! When we understand how the brain makes habits, we can easily and quickly create new habits and replace old ones. To understand habits, we need to understand the brain in finer detail. The brain is made up of a neural net – millions of brain cells wired together. Neurons are cells in the brain that connect with other cells through synapses. These connections are like a hand with many fingers. The fingers can con-

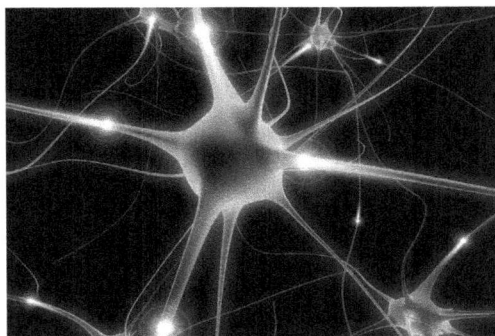

Image of a neuron and its connectors to other neurons, chains of which set up neural pathways

nect with the fingers of other neurons.

This is how the brain learns; it actually makes new connections between neurons and creates pathways. The neurons that fire together more often become preferred pathways; when triggered, these neuronal pathways will fire first – automatically.

A habit is simply a learned pathway that has linked neurons; over time and with repetition these pathways then become automatic.

Repetition is the key that turns a thought, a feeling, or a behavior into a habit.

We've all heard the old saying, "It takes 30 days to make a new habit." Well, that idea is simply outdated. What is happening is really repetition. During the course of the 30 days, we're adding something to our routine consistently and repeatedly until it becomes a preferred pathway in the brain.

Changing a habit can be as simple as learning something new. We are learning new things all the time. With the tools of NLP, we can set up a new pathway in the brain, condense the repetition, and turn it to a new habit very quickly. We no longer need 30 days to make a new habit.

In understanding our habits, we have triggers or cues that tell the brain when to run the habit. The following story illustrates a simple habit and the awareness of my trigger behind it.

Understanding Triggers

When I moved to Portland, Oregon, I wanted to make chocolate chip cookies all the time. Every day I was getting the feeling, the craving to make cookies. It wasn't just about eating cookies; it was about the whole process of making them. I had piles of cookies, and after a few weeks my pants started getting tighter.

After shopping for larger pants, finally I asked myself, "Why do I want to make cookies all the time?"

As I gave it some quiet reflection, childhood memories started coming to mind. It was dark and stormy outside, all five of us kids were laughing and talking in a warm, cozy kitchen while making and eating chocolate chip cookies.

I grew up in Utah where it is almost always sunny. Even when it snows, the sun still shines through. The days it rained were few but intense. The skies were dark and stormy, thunder crashed across the sky, and the rains were torrential. These were the days we stayed inside and made chocolate chip cookies.

That would have been fine for Utah, but then I moved to Portland, Oregon. Portland is about as rainy as Utah is sunny.

From my history growing up in Utah, my brain had created the association of rain and making chocolate chip cookies. So every time it rained my brain said, "It's cookie time!" and I would get the craving to make cookies. Rain was my trigger, the cue telling my brain when to run the cookie habit.

Our habits can range from simple to complex. The simplest level is an association like cookies and rain. Sometimes, just the awareness of the habit is enough to change it. I no longer have to make cookies every time it rains (thank goodness, or I'd be in trouble).

Assessing Your Habits and Triggers

The first part of changing habits is to identify what the habits are. What are the habits that are getting in your way of healthy living and releasing weight?

And, now, thinking of your habits, what is the trigger, the cue that tells your brain when to run the habit?

One of the ladies in class, we'll call her Susan, identified what was going on for her. "There is a certain co-worker, that every time I talk to her, I need to go out and find the donut cart. My communication with her makes me feel small and belittled. Finding the donut cart has been my way of reaching for comfort after talking with her."

Layers of Habits: Associations, Meanings

The simplest level of a habit is an association, like my association of rainy days and making cookies. Another example comes from the famous story of Pavlov and his dogs. Pavlov was a psychology researcher who worked with dogs; he always rang a bell before he fed his dogs their dinner. Pavlov noticed that after awhile the dogs would salivate as soon as they heard the bell. The dogs had created the association between the sound of the bell and food, and salivation was an automatic response because in their minds they made the connection that the bell meant food.

In a way we are all like Pavlov's dogs; we all have a history of food associations. Our foods have history, and from this history foods take on meanings. For example, what do you think of when you think of pumpkin pie or apple pie?

Because of how our brain learns and our ability to make associations, the present moment is never just about the present moment; it's about our whole history connected to it. For example, a hot fudge sundae is not just frozen sweet milk and chocolate goo, it's really connected with every time mom or dad sat down with you over a sundae, or every time your grades were rewarded with a sundae, or every social event that included sundaes.

Our foods have history and meanings attached to them.

Your food choices, preferences, and cravings are really about your past programs and the history connected to them. You have been conditioned to like the foods you enjoy.

If you lived in the typical American home, you may have grown up with food rewards. Perhaps you got a candy bar for good behavior or you went out for ice cream when you got good grades. The unconscious mind tracks all these meanings and history connected with food and sums them up into a feeling. And now as an adult, when you want to feel rewarded you typically reach for the same foods you were rewarded with as a kid-and these food associations are also connected to feelings and cravings.

Your Food History, Associations, Meanings

To begin identifying your food associations, start by thinking of your food habits and cravings. Next, identify the associations and meanings connected to those foods and cravings.

When you were rewarded as a kid, what kinds of rewards were you given?

_____

_____

_____

Do you have certain foods that mean celebration or social connection?

_____

_____

_____

What foods mean comfort? What foods mean stress relief?

_____

_____

_____

What other meanings are connected with foods and your food habits?

_____

_____

_____

Think of the habits you listed earlier. What meanings are connected to these habits?

_____

_____

_____

Create New Associations

One of the simplest ways to change your food meanings is to create new associations. In NLP terms it is referred to as changing sub modalities. We can change how we perceive foods by changing the qualities we associate with them.

For this example, I am going to use a bowl of chips. When we think of a food, we have a visual image of it and the qualities associated with the mental picture; we also have mental representations of the other senses as well: what we hear, feel, smell, and taste. You'll notice how your brain represents the chips, and by changing these mental representations, you can also change your feelings about them.

NLP Tool: Changing the Mental Pictures

Step 1: Imagine a bowl of chips in front of you. Notice how you picture it in your mind: Is it in color? Is it three dimensional? Notice what you like about the chips; is it the flavor, texture, sight, sound of the crunch?

Step 2: On a scale of 1 to 10, if the bowl of chips were in front of you now, how compelled would you feel to eat them (10 being high that you couldn't pass them up; 1 being no desire for them)?

Step 3: Now change your mental pictures and help your mind create new associations. Imagine picking up a chip, biting into it, crunching it, and noticing it tastes a little off. Then you notice it tastes gritty, like sand gritting against your teeth – yuck! Spit it out. Blah!

Step 4: Now notice the bowl of chips on a scale of 1 to 10. How tempting are the chips now?

Step 5: Now imagine all the color draining out of the bowl of chips so both bowl and chips turn black and white.

Step 6: On a scale of 1 to 10, how tempting are they now? Notice what has changed in your feeling about them.

The chips become less compelling the more we change the mental experience. This is one way to create new associations and mental habits. We can change the qualities of each of the senses, for example the quality of the visual picture, the quality of the sounds or the feel and texture, or the quality of the taste or the smell.

Repetition is key: The mental imagery process is now stored in your "chips" file. The next time you see a bowl of chips, your unconscious mind will review everything in the chips file and give you a feeling about it. As it sums up the history, it sums up your experience (even imagined experience) and you end up with a feeling. Going through this process five or more times will help your brain wire in a new association (or new neural pathway) for chips.

Note: I recommend staying away from negative imagery and using it only for those foods that are obviously very un-healthy. We still want to be able to enjoy our food; we just want to change our unhealthy patterns with food.

Replace Old Habits by Creating New Associations

In some cases, replacing an old habit is as simple as remembering a new behavior. The next exercise offers a way of training your mind to create a new habit. We will use mental cues that "remind" you to replace the old habit with what you'd rather be doing.

In replacing a habit, we first must identify the cues or triggers that tell the mind when to run the old habit. For instance, if you have been conditioned to clean your plate, then you don't get the cue to stop eating until your plate is clean. So, the cue to stop eating becomes seeing a clean plate rather than your body noticing when you are full. Even if you are stuffed, you may feel compelled to squeeze in those last few bites.

The Clean Plate Club is very common. Parents taught us to clean our plates for a variety of positive reasons. In most cases they were well meaning and just wanted to make sure their kids had enough to eat and got the nourishment growing bodies needed. Other positive reasons included appreciating food, minimizing waste, and feeling gratitude.

After years of making sure I cleaned my plate, the "I'm full" signal to stop eating was suppressed. Making sure my plate was clean became the cue to stop eating. (Until I realized and changed this cue, buffets were brutal, seriously brutal). However, cleaning the plate is just a mental habit, and now we have the tools to change it. All brain habits are simply what we've learned, and we can always learn something new.

I knew I no longer wanted to be compelled to clean my plate. I would rather notice when I am full and satisfied and find it easy to stop eating when I reached the point of being comfortably full.

When you've identified what you would rather be doing instead of cleaning your plate, you simply need practice and repetition for the mind to automate it. But rather than taking 30 days to run through it every day while focusing conscious attention on every meal, you can simply repeat it several times in your mind and create new mental cues – new mental pathways-that will replace the old behavior.

If you've been part of the Clean Plate Club, use this exercise to help your mind learn new cues about when to stop eating and what to do instead. This process is a variation on the NLP Swish pattern, which uses a pattern interrupt sequence.

Break Free of the Clean Your Plate Club

In your mind's eye, imagine that you are sitting down to dinner. You have a beautiful plate of healthy food in front of you and you begin to enjoy your meal. See yourself in your typical dinner environment with the people around you whom you usually see.

When you've finished about three-quarters of your food, you begin to notice that you feel full, even noticing a wonderful feeling of satisfaction. Looking at your plate, notice that the food looks less appealing and you feel like eating less and less. You might even hear yourself thinking, I'm done. You also might notice yourself eating slower, and you notice you would rather keep that wonderful feeling of being comfortably full rather than feeling stuffed.

Way off in the distance, you notice a bright spark. It begins to come closer and closer, faster and faster, until it explodes in front of you into a big refrigerator. You realize it's so easy to wrap up and save the rest of your food for later (preserving the intention of not wasting food), or if you are in a restaurant, you can box it up and take it with you, and you can still enjoy it later.

Imagine automatically getting up from your dinner, wrapping it up, and putting it away in the refrigerator while you feel so comfortably satisfied. By stopping eating when you feel satisfied and comfortably full, you can appreciate your meal that much more as you focus on the feeling of being so satisfied.

This brief visualization used some mental cues for breaking the old Clean Plate Club habit. To get your mind to make this response automatic, repeat this exercise five to eight times; your mind will begin to create a new thought pattern and a new habit of noticing when you are comfortably full. After you've repeated it enough, you'll notice that it's natural to stop eating when you are full rather than needing to clean your plate.

Notice that the next time you sit down to dinner you pay more attention to the feeling of being comfortably full as a cue to stop eating rather than having to finish your plate. In your mind, you are telling your brain what you want it to do and then running through the new pattern several times.

All your brain needs is repetition to turn your new thought pattern into a habit. And your new habit will run automatically even without you consciously thinking about it once it is incorporated into your autopilot system.

In the next chapter, we will look at emotional drivers-the underlying patterns behind habits-and how to change them. But first let's take a look at other mental habits that could be working against you.

Stress Habits

Just as we have habits in our thoughts and feelings, we can also have stress habits in our brain, when our body goes into a stress response when we encounter a trigger. When we experience stress, our body responds by activating the fight or flight response in our nervous system.

Our nervous system has two pathways that work opposite each other. The stress mode is the *fight or flight* response; the relax mode is the *rest and digest* response. When our body is operating in fight or flight mode, it stops the activity of rest and digest, and vice versa.

When our body is in rest and digest mode, it focuses on digestion and absorption of food and boosting our immune function, blood is directed to our organs for digestion. When our body is in fight or flight mode, it prepares to fight off an attacker or run away. Blood is moved to the muscles and the body releases stress hormones – adrenaline and cortisol – which prepare the body for fight or flight and give it access to quick physical energy.

The fight or flight response was more useful to us in ancient times when we had physical threats that needed immediate physical responses, but think of the things that cause us stress now:

- Co-workers

- Family relationships

- Money concerns

- Job performance

- Ornery customers

- Bad attitudes

• Traffic

Most of the stressors we encounter now are not life threatening and a physical response is inappropriate. So, if a co-worker criticizes us at work, we just take it, sitting in our chemical stew of adrenaline and cortisol. As our body goes through the stress response on the inside, we can maintain a calm outer appearance that is a more socially acceptable behavior.

Do you eat when you are stressed? Eating when we are stressed is one way to feel more calm because it engages the rest and digest response, but it can cause us to gain weight and eventually leads to more stress.

If we have elevated levels of the stress hormone cortisol over time and the levels aren't normalizing, it can actually cause us to gain weight, eat more, and retain extra body fat. With the increase of stress in our lives, it becomes increasingly important to find ways to help the mind and body de-stress.

By giving your mind some new associations for relaxing, you can help your brain change the stress habits that lead to stress eating, elevated cortisol, and thus weight gain. Having positive strategies for de-stressing are important to helping your body normalize and function at its best.

Exercise is a great way to help the body de-stress because it gives the body the physical release for which the fight or flight response prepares us. Other de-stress activities include relaxing to music, journaling, having quiet time, positive social time with family or friends, yoga, stretching, and doing activities you love and enjoy.

Make time to relax; have some time during your day that allows you to de-stress. Even a 10 minute walk during your lunch hour is a great way to get the mind and body to release stress, get a break from work, and refocus your mind.

The other part of stress reduction is how our brain handles stress. You may know some people who handle stress very well and others who don't seem to handle stress at all. The difference is in their perception of the situation, their stress habits, and the mental patterns behind how the body responds.

Most stressors we experience now are perceived threats. It's how we think about the stressors that determine how stressed we get. If I have a mental habit of thinking "What is the worst that can happen?" my mind could easily be caught up in continuous stress. This is a pattern I see with my anxiety clients; their brains are sorting for the worst case scenario.

To help the mind change the stress habits even before they start, we can work at the brain level. By practicing breathing paired with calming cues, we can set up a new habit to reduce the mental stress and feel more comfortable and confident in stressful situations.

Here is a brief example of a mindfulness exercise. Even taking 5-10 minutes to sit quietly and move your awareness through your body can help your mind and body system relax and de-stress. (This exercise is also available as the recording "Train Your Brain for Stress Relief," available through my website.)

As you go through this exercise, focus on your breath and being comfortable in your body. As you feel calm and comfortable, your mind is connecting the relaxation and the breathing along with the visuals you use. Then, when you find you are in a stressful situation, you can use the same breathing, breathing through your body, or using the visual of the bubble, and your body will respond with the relaxation response. The more you practice it, the easier your body will step into it.

Mindfulness Exercise

Sit back, get comfortable, and begin by taking a couple of deep relaxing breaths. Let the breath fill your lungs; hold the breath at the top of your lungs. Imagine gathering all the stress and tension of the day. Focus it into your lungs and release it as you exhale. Take in another deep and gentle breath, allowing it to fill your lungs, once again, gathering out all the stress and tension from your body, focusing it into your lungs, and releasing it as you exhale. You can allow your mind and body to feel more and more relaxed, more focused with every breath.

Now, imagine breathing in with your next breath and focusing your awareness on just the bottoms of your feet, paying attention to the bottoms of your feet, how they feel inside your shoes, and release the breath. With the next breath, breathing in, moving your awareness up through your feet into your left ankle, paying attention to the left ankle and how that feels and releasing the breath. With your next breath, moving your attention up to the awareness of your right knee and focusing on how your right knee feels against your pants. With your next breath, moving your awareness up to your left thigh, breathing in gently and feeling so relaxed and focused in the present moment.

With your next breath, breathing in your awareness into your stomach and notice how your stomach feels. Breathing in with your next breath, move your awareness up into your chest. With your next breath, moving your awareness to your heart; you may even notice the rhythm of your heart beating. With your next breath, breathe your awareness up into your throat. With your next breath, move your awareness through your body and into your head.

Feel what it's like to be here now in the present moment while feeling calm and comfortable and so relaxed. You might even imagine the feeling of being comfortable and relaxed surrounding you like a bubble. Feel what it's like to be so comfortable and relaxed inside your bubble; even though the outside world is busy, you can remain comfortable and relaxed. Your mind can be focused and clear and your body can be relaxed.

This exercise brings your awareness to being in your body and focusing in the present moment. By bringing your awareness and attention back to the present moment, you can feel more calm and focused rather than speculating about problems in the future. When we worry, it's as if our mind is off somewhere in the future, making up stories about what might happen.

You can even use a breathing cue to help your mind and body make the connection for relaxing, just by thinking about breathing through your body and feeling calm and relaxed. I like using the image of a bubble; it gives your mind a visual cue to focus on and will help you feel calm and relaxed when you think about it. By using internal cues for relaxing, you can access this feeling of being relaxed just by thinking about the cues you paired with it, such as the breathing or visuals like the bubble.

Now, think about a situation when you would normally feel stress. Imagine breathing through your body and letting yourself feel that calm and comfortable way of feeling; picturing the bubble of calm around you, imagine stepping into that situation and notice how you feel differently.

You can remain calm and comfortable and your body can be relaxed even in situations that require you to respond quickly. By using this mindfulness exercise, the visualizations and breathing, you can train your mind and body to remain calm and yet focused in different situations, allowing you to think more clearly and even handle the situations better.

When the body goes into the stress response, it actually limits the blood to the brain as the body moves the blood to the muscles for quick action. This is one reason that logic seems to go out the window when we are stressed. As our mind stays focused and the body remains calm, we are better able to access logic and reasoning, allowing us to better handle the stressful situation.

As your mind learns to relax, your body also follows and can balance and normalize your stress hormones more effectively. Your mind can be focused and yet your body can be calm and relaxed. This combination is actually ideal for the stressors we encounter today, which require us to be level-headed and re-main calm.

Make Positive Mental Habits

Many of us tend to have negative habits regarding how we see ourselves. For example, when you look in a mirror, what do you think? You might notice your imperfections or focus on what you don't like.

Think of the times you've been criticized or belittled. How do you feel when you are criticized? It makes us shrink back, feel small and withdrawn as well as resentful toward the criti-cizer. Some criticisms we say to ourselves we wouldn't dream of saying to others.

Criticism saps our energy and causes us to feel down or depressed. Criticism breeds resentment. It's time to stop criti-cizing ourselves and others! Let it stop here with you!

You can be your own worst enemy-or our own best friend. Which are you?

Often, we criticize and belittle ourselves and then expect ourselves to be motivated even though we've just undercut our own efforts. If we are creating self-resentment through criticism, we are destroying our own motivation. If we want to find more motivation and enthusiasm for the changes we are making, we need to stay focused on the positives.

Think of the times you were encouraged, supported, and appreciated for your efforts. When we are encouraged and appreciated, we feel good and so we are more motivated to do more; we are even excited and enthused. We stand a little taller, feel more positive, and are inspired to reach out beyond our old comfort zone.

When we praise and appreciate others, we believe in them and ask the best from them-and that's what we get back in return! It's time to change how we see ourselves and create some new habits of appreciation, love, and awe.

Use Appreciation for Motivation

Notice what you are doing well, appreciate yourself and your body, and you will have more fuel for staying on track and motivated. To connect with the positive emotions you are truly looking for, you don't have to do anything; you can feel them even as quickly as thinking about them.

The next exercise uses the understanding of anchors from NLP plus engages the positive emotions of appreciation, love, and awe. This exercise comes from self-actualization psychologist, L. Michael Hall, author of Secrets of Personal Mastery. It is a great tool to create a new habit of feeling good about yourself so you can be positive and stay motivated.

By using some simple principles, we can help the brain set up a trigger or new association. We do this by pairing a feeling from a memory with visualizing and touching three places on the arm. When we've set the anchor (the touch), we can access it anytime to bring up the positive feeling-even instantly!

The premise of this process is just like conditioning, a psychological term meaning our brain pairs things together, creating an association. In this case we use our own memories to access a feeling and we use a touch cue to trigger it at will.

NLP Tool: Anchoring Appreciation, Love and Awe

Think of three different things that inspire the feelings of appreciation, love, and awe. Pick something that you appreciate, something that you love, and a time or place when you felt awe. Good examples of awe include standing on top of a mountain overlooking a vista, on the shore of the ocean, or other beautiful scenes in nature. Create visuals for each one.

Appreciation: _____

_____

Love: _____

_____

Awe: _____

_____

Next, set up the anchors or triggers. Using the first finger of your right hand as a pointer, touch your left arm first at the wrist, second touch at the halfway point between the wrist and elbow, and the third point is to touch above the elbow.

Setting the Anchors: Pair the touch and the feeling together, think of appreciation while holding the touch 3-5 seconds. Pairing the touch and thought together helps the brain make the association between the touch and the thought or feeling. Release the anchor when the feeling is at its strongest.

Step 1: As you touch your wrist, think of the thing you appreciate. See it out in front of you. Let that wonderful feeling of appreciation wash over you from your head to your toes, and let that feeling get stronger and stronger. You may even imagine a dial in your mind so you can turn up the feeling. Release the touch when the feeling is at its strongest.

Step 2: Next, touch your arm halfway between your wrist and elbow and think of the thing that you love. Imagine seeing it out in front of you and let that wave of love pour over you. Let that wonderful feeling of love wash over you from your head to your toes, and let that feeling get stronger and stronger. You may even imagine a dial so you can turn up the feeling. Release the touch when the feeling is at its strongest.

Step 3: Then, touch the crook of your arm above your elbow and think of the time and place that you felt awe. Imagine being there now, see what you were seeing, hear what you were hearing, and let the feeling pour through you. Let the feeling get stronger and stronger. Turn up your imaginary dial, and release the touch when the feeling is at its strongest.

Break State: Now, look around the room for a couple seconds, which tells the mind the process is complete. Then, test the anchors you set.

Test the anchor: Touch each of the same places on your arm (engaging the anchors) and recall the feelings that are now associated with each place. Notice how your brain has connected the touch and the feeling.

Step 4: Touching the place at your wrist (first anchor), think of the thing you appreciate and let that wonderful feeling wash over you. Now, simply apply it to yourself. Let the wave of appreciation wash through you and bring to your awareness all that you appreciate about you. Let yourself bask in that wonderful feeling of appreciation for yourself; let that feeling grow stronger and stronger.

Step 5: Touching your arm between your wrist and elbow (second anchor), think of the thing you love and let the feeling of love wash over you from your head to your toes. Let the feeling of love pour through you and now simply apply it to yourself, letting it wash through you. It feels so good to feel love for yourself, doesn't it?

Step 6: Touching your arm above the elbow, think of the time you felt awe (third anchor). Let the feeling of awe wash over you, and now simply apply it to yourself, letting it wash through you. The feeling of awe applied to the self might feel a little strange, but let's focus on just one of the body's amazing systems that work to keep us living and breathing with health and well-being.

Taking in a deep breath, let it fill your lungs; be aware that all the air filling your lungs is filtering down into the lung's tiny membranes. The blood moves across those membranes, and the tiny molecules of air are filtering across, being picked up by the blood and carried to all parts of your body, to every tissue and every organ system, where the blood releases the oxygen and picks up the carbon dioxide to bring it back to your lungs and you release it as you exhale.

Thinking of just one body system-your lungs and the air that flows through you-your body is truly amazing. Your body keeps all your cells and tissues working so harmoniously with every breath you take-and it does it automatically! You are amazed at your body aren't you? Feel the awe for your amazing body and then let the awe wash over you, from your head to your toes, simply applying it to yourself. Isn't it amazing to be you?

Let the feelings of appreciation, love, and awe inspire you!

Any time you use these touches or anchors, your brain will recall these feelings. You can connect with any feeling you want even as simply as you think about it. The more you practice, the easier it becomes as your brain reinforces the new habit of positive feelings.

If you use this anchor process while you look at yourself in the mirror, you can set up a positive mental habit of appreciation for yourself. So many of us have negative mental habits and pick ourselves apart when we see our reflections in the mirror. What if you felt appreciated, loved, and even felt awe for being alive each time you saw yourself in the mirror! It would feel so great, wouldn't it?

Now that you have set up the anchor, you can do this exercise in front of the mirror. Go through the sequence, feel the feelings, and use the touches; let the wonderful feelings pour through you as you see your reflection in the mirror. Your brain will begin to connect these wonderful feelings with your reflection-and wouldn't that be a much better habit?

I also recommend posting notes that remind you to appreciate, love, and feel awe for who you are. Why wait to appreciate yourself when you are thinner? Chances are you were thinner before and you didn't appreciate yourself then. Begin by feeling better about yourself now!

Just as we respond to appreciation from others, we also respond to the appreciation we offer ourselves. Why wait for others to give us the positive feelings we crave? We can connect with appreciation, love, and awe instantly!

Though the reasons for hanging onto extra weight may vary from person to person, a common reason for gaining weight is that we feel blocked from the feelings of love and appreciation. For example, if I am craving comfort foods, the craving often stems from an underlying feeling of not feeling loved or supported.

As you appreciate and love yourself more, you release the inner struggle and can allow the process of releasing the weight to be easier and more natural. Besides, it just feels better to feel appreciation, love, and awe rather than criticism, and these positive feelings will fuel your motivation.

If loving and appreciating who you are is a challenge for you, use disc #3, "Enlighten Your Body Image," in *A Lighter You! Mind Body Weight Loss* CD set. It helps you visualize releasing old labels and setting up new mental habits in how you see yourself. Plus, it will help you internalize a sense of comfort and wellbeing so that you do not need to find comfort from food.

Chapter 3: Transform Cravings and Addictions

Willpower Is Not Enough

Have you ever said, "I am going to stop eating sugar" and then suddenly it's as if you see it everywhere? It's like sugar begins jumping out at you and things you wouldn't normally notice draw your attention, as if the bakery items are taunting you and you can almost hear them laughing at you like schoolchildren. You may pass up the first cookie, feel pretty good about yourself, pass up the soda – but then the doughnut comes along and you give in.

This isn't just about sugar; it applies to any habit, craving, or addiction, including smoking, drinking, and even drug use. When you set your mind to avoid something, you spend a lot of time and energy trying to avoid it.

What we focus on grows. If we focus on the problem, guess what? The problem becomes bigger, if only in our mind.

Remember learning in Chapter One that we need to focus on the positive? When you make up your mind to avoid something, you are actually setting your mind to notice it more because of how your unconscious mind interprets your words.

Try saying the phrase "I'm not going to eat sugar." What do you think of with this phrase? That's right – sugar. Avoidance simply fuels the problem with more power. If you are using the strategy of avoiding a temptation, you will have to plan your life around avoiding it.

We don't want to keep avoiding things that get in our way; we want to create healthy boundaries with them instead. It's even better if we face and transform the problem; then we can be more in control of our choices and our lives.

To stop struggling with cravings or addictions, you must engage your deeper awareness and address what is *driving* the behavior – the mental and emotional patterns. Cravings are a feeling that comes from our deeper awareness, even from our unconscious mind.

In the old method of changing a habit, we would identify what we want – "I want to stop eating chocolate" – and then try to stick to it. We may be good for a few days, but then after a few more days we might give in to the old cravings and fall off the wagon. We experience it as a struggle with ourselves. It's as if a part of us wants to change and a part of us doesn't.

But, that's not all, we then berate ourselves thinking, "If only I was more disciplined, I could make myself do it." But discipline means making ourselves do something we didn't want to do in the first place. I would rather work from positive motivation than from discipline.

In working with addictions or with changing habits, the principles are the same. Rather than setting a goal and just trying to stick to it, we can shine the light of awareness onto old behaviors to transform them into something new and more supportive.

When changing old habits, it is especially important to notice the cue or trigger and what is driving the behavior. If we don't take care of the *emotional driver*, the emotion behind the behavior or the habit, it will find a new expression. Without addressing the underlying emotional driver, we may substitute one bad habit for another. You may know someone who quit smoking, only to take up nervous snacking and so gained weight.

When we understand the underlying patterns behind the behavior, we can bring together the part of us that wants to change and the part of us that doesn't for a new purpose. By aligning these parts of ourselves, we reduce the internal conflict and thus end the struggle. All the energy that went into the old behavior can now be harnessed to help us stay on track with what we really want.

What if you could take all that energy you express as a craving and direct it to help you stay motivated, eat healthier, or even crave fruits and vegetables? Well, now you can and I'll show you how.

The following story comes from a client and is a great illustration of how to identify what is connected to cravings and addictions. The name has been changed but the story is real, and in just one session we changed what would have been labeled an addiction by using NLP tools and strategies of alignment.

Alcoholic No More

Roger came to see me because he wanted to use his time more effectively. I asked him, "What are you doing now and what would you like to do differently?"

Roger said, "Well, when I get home from work I usually have four or five beers, and then I don't get anything done. I wouldn't say I have a drinking problem. I'm not addicted, but I just want to use my time better."

I asked, "Roger, would it be okay to go a week without a drink?" A grimace passed over his face.

He said, "I could do it, but I just wouldn't choose to and it certainly wouldn't be comfortable. But, if I could drink less, maybe I could be more motivated to pursue other things that would improve my life, such as better health and being more motivated to work on my business."

I directed Roger in the NLP process called Hands Polarity. "Holding your hands out in front of you, let one hand represent the part of you that holds the problem (drinking) and the other hand represent the change you want (stop drinking)."

I turned his attention to the hand that represented drinking and asked the golden question: "What does this behavior get for you?"

He thought for a moment, introspecting, and then said, "Courage."

Drinking was Roger's way for connecting with courage. Courage can be very positive, but in the impaired state of inebriation, courage can become misdirected and inappropriate. Roger had related some stories when his behavior while drinking had been a little over the top, even destructive.

I asked, "This part in charge of drinking, would it be willing to connect with courage in other ways rather than only through drinking?"

Roger answered, "Yes."

I asked, "Roger, in what other activities do you find a feeling of courage?"

He thought a moment and then realized, "When I work out, I have that feeling of confidence and courage."

I continued, "Would it be okay if this part were in charge of getting you to go to the gym and work out as a method of connecting with courage?"

Roger reflected a moment, feeling for the answer, and then said, "Yes comes to mind."

"Great. Now turn your attention to the hand that wants to quit drinking. What does this part want for you?"

"More motivation to work on my business and to use my time better," he said.

"Now have both of these parts look over and appreciate what each of them wants for you-the part in charge of drinking and the part that wants to quit. How does each part feel to be acknowledged and appreciated for what each is trying to do for you?"

He moved the palms of his hands to face each other. "Good, it feels like they are acknowledged and heard."

"Now, looking to the future you are even now creating, how can both of these parts work together to create what you really want-that healthy life that is working for you, full of motivation, moving your life forward with health, happiness, and success?"

"Well, instead of going home and drinking, I see myself reading books to better myself, I am going to the gym and working out, and I am focusing on building my business," he said.

"As these two parts of you are now working together, what more do you see for yourself?"

"I see more motivation, more focus, more energy from going to the gym. I can use my time for improving my life, moving my life forward and living better."

"What is an image or symbol that represents courage for you?" I asked.

"A lion."

"Now, imagine taking that image of a lion and shrinking it down, and notice where you would like to keep that image with you so that you know you are always connected to courage."

"Hmm, I guess in my heart," he said.

"Wonderful, now as both of these parts can see how they can work together for this positive healthy future and the part of you that used to drink for courage now has a new focus, we are going to ask your unconscious mind to begin moving your hands together, but only as quickly as you are able to increase the communication and connection between these two parts of you."

Roger's hands started to move together just a couple of inches. Then he stopped and said, "Well, if I give up drinking completely, I will miss out on some good parties, I don't want to miss out."

(This is an underlying objection that is very important to address in the process so internal alignment can be created.)

"So, if courage were integrated into your life and you wouldn't need to drink to connect with courage, what would drinking be about for you instead?" I asked.

He thought a moment. "I guess relaxing and enjoying the social scene."

"Great. So if you can still enjoy social drinking, not as a way of expressing courage because you already have that but as a way of relaxing and enjoying the social scene, would that be okay?" I asked.

He thought a moment while he was feeling for the answer. "Well, yes."

Roger's hands continued to move toward each other over the next couple of minutes until his hands came together and interlaced.

I asked, "As you look at your evenings now, reading books and working on your business rather than drinking, how does it look to you?"

"It looks doable, even easy, and I feel motivated to get working on my business," Roger said.

The next week when Roger came in, he was flabbergasted. He said, "This is so amazing! When I went home from work the next day I started a beer, but I didn't even want to finish it. It just didn't appeal to me."

So, in a single session Roger no longer had a "drinking problem." By asking the part of his mind in charge of drinking to redirect its focus in line with what he really wanted, he gave it a new job and created internal alignment.

If Roger had gone through the self-denial and discipline route, given up drinking cold turkey, a part of him would have felt as if he were giving up his connection to courage. However, by giving the *positive feelings* to the part in charge of the old behavior, he could tap into courage in other ways and move forward with ease. Rather than needing an external action (drinking) to connect with courage, we set up an internal cue (the lion image) for Roger to connect with courage.

In Roger's mind, if he were to give up drinking he would be giving up courage unless he found a new source for courage.

Rather than fighting against himself, trying to suppress cravings, trying to avoid drinking, or spending years with a label of being an addict, this process allowed his unconscious mind to shift its focus and the problem transformed. Once his unconscious mind had a new focus and outlet for courage, Roger was now free to focus his energy on other things. He could even still enjoy light social drinking when he wanted.

The problem transformed because he changed the meaning connected to it.

Drinking just didn't have the appeal it had before because the underlying meaning changed.

A common perception is that we are at war with anything we don't like. We fight cancer and disease, we have declared war on drugs, but these problems only get bigger. We fight with ourselves trying to control cravings, but because we focus on the problems, they get larger.

As the problems get larger we feel more out of control and less able to change. Will power alone doesn't work, and it often has a backlash. As we try to deny what we want and even cut off the part of us that wants it, we perpetuate internal conflict.

Then somewhere along the line our culture labels the problem a disease. Then we no longer have control; we place it in the hands of the medical community and it's as if there is nothing we can do about it. We might as well give up unless there is a pill to "fix" it.

When we assume a label, we assume a whole set of problems that may not even be ours. Along with a label comes all the baggage that has been associated with the problem for other people. After we've labeled something, the problem becomes much bigger than just the behavior. When we call something a disease, there is a sense that it is out of our hands and so beyond our control, but it is still under the control of our *unconscious mind.*

Cravings and addictions are rooted in our history and come from our unconscious mind and the meanings connected to them. Because it is our unconscious mind at work, they are not logical and rational, and mostly, we just notice the feeling or compulsion. If we continue to focus on changing just the behavior, we will continue to struggle. The cravings and addictions represent a part of our unconscious mind that wants something positive - a feeling. Even though we identify the behavior as negative like overeating or cravings, the underlying desire is for a positive feeling and that part of us wants to be heard. It's why willpower has a backlash: the more we try to suppress it, the harder that part of us fights back.

However, if we make a simple paradigm shift and see all our behaviors and cravings as *symptoms* pointing to a deeper issue, we can understand the deeper patterns that are driving our lives. Rather than perpetuating a war within ourselves, we can engage our deeper awareness and evolve the habits, the cravings, and the addictions to find a better pathway of expression. Most often it's about allowing ourselves to connect with these positive feelings in healthy ways.

Rather than fighting ourselves, we can work with our awareness to engage our own energies for moving forward. Rather than focusing on just changing the behavior, it's even more important to look for what the behavior represents. Then, we can give that part of us the positive feeling it is looking for, in Roger's case it was courage.

In Chapter Two we went through the simple NLP tool of anchoring appreciation, love, and awe. We can access any feeling we want just by thinking about it. In Roger's example, he internalized the feeling of courage and gave the part a different expression of courage which then took care of the emotional driver, and so the behavior was no longer a problem.

In NLP terms we see addiction not as a disease but as a *learned* behavior and a symptom pointing to a deeper issue. Whether its alcohol, food, smoking, or even drug use, no matter the addiction, the principles are the same. We've attached a meaning to the habit (or the outcome) and the behavior is about what the unconscious mind thinks the habit will get for us - a feeling.

Now, some people might say that the brain of an addict is different from the normal brain, so addiction must be a disease. It is true that the brain operates differently for an addict, but this brings up the question: Which came first, the chicken or the egg?

Did the brain become an addicted brain because it was destined to, or did the person think a series of thoughts and engage in a series of behaviors that over time developed into mental habits and feelings and eventually formed the brain pattern we label an "addicted" brain?

Mental habits, old patterns, and feelings are within our ability to change, but we need a new approach.

The problem is not the behavior as much as what is driving the behavior and what it represents to us. Weight problems are only a symptom; by understanding what weight represents, we can more quickly transform the problem.

If we address the underlying meanings, use our inner awareness to refocus the part of us in charge of the behavior, we can adopt new behaviors and strategies – and the problem transforms!

Let's keep it simple! Unwanted behaviors, even if they are automatic, are simply behaviors and something we've learned. It sounds much easier to change a habit or behavior than an addiction, doesn't it? That's because of all the meanings we've attached to the word addiction, we assume it's out of our control or that it must be really hard and take a lot of work and that we will always struggle with it.

But, we have a lot of experience in changing old habits. They are something we've learned, and we can learn something new. In fact, we are learning new things all the time, and our brain creates new neuronal pathways with the new things we learn.

As we open our awareness to understanding ourselves, we can address our habits, cravings, and even addictions with wisdom rather than battling against ourselves.

By engaging our inner wisdom and working with the part of us in charge of the behavior rather than against it, we will find it much easier to make the change and keep it. The part of us in charge of the old behavior, the part that doesn't want to change, is still trying to get something positive for us. Recognize and acknowledge this part and give it access to what it really wants- the positive feeling-and the negative behavior transforms.

Every part of us is trying to get something positive. Usually it's about a feeling, and we can connect with positive feelings just by thinking about them.

By working with a new focus for alignment, we no longer need to fight against ourselves or deny the part of us we don't like. This new approach engages our wisdom and transforms the behavior through compassion and awareness.

By addressing these challenges with insight and wisdom, we can embrace our whole selves in moving forward on the journey of life. Change can be easy and fun as we pay attention to our deeper awareness and motivations. We have access to all the positive feelings we've ever felt, and we can access them as quickly as we think about them. We can simply shift the focus of the negatives and create alignment with the life we really want.

Note: This brief example of one person's experience in no way means that other people struggling with alcohol are seeking courage, but rather it illustrates that each individual has associations, meanings, and history represented through a habit or addiction. In Roger's case the association was fairly simple. The underlying reasons and meanings vary and are unique to each person. Depending on the person's history, the associations may be more complex and even involve deeply held beliefs, which we will address in Chapter Five.

Assessing Your Emotional Drivers

Think of the habits you identified earlier. You can find the emotional driver by asking the part of you in charge of the habit, "What do you want?" This question will help you find new levels of the answer. In the example of my chocolate chip cookie habit, I was the queen cookie maker, I had the chocolate chip cookie recipe memorized by the time I was in second grade. Whenever I made cookies, I was the center of attention, and everyone would gather around me, for me those memories also represented being connected to my family. When I made chocolate chip cookies, I was remembering at the unconscious level the feelings of comfort and connection.

We don't have to rely on the habit to bring the feeling to us; we can connect with the feeling in other ways. I began to call my family, staying connected with them by phone rather than waiting for the crisis impulse of cookies.

To truly transform a craving, habit, or addiction, we must replace the emotional driver.

Emotional Drivers Assessment

List your habits or cravings on the left and then ask, "What is that trying to get for me?" That will point to your emotional drivers.

Habits and Cravings   **The Emotional Drivers**

_____   _____

_____   _____

_____   _____

_____   _____

_____   _____

Ask yourself, "What do I really want?"

The next time you find yourself doing the old habit, ask yourself, "What do I *really* want?" This is a great question to post on your refrigerator. Whenever you find yourself headed for a snack, if you ask yourself "What do I really want?" you'll begin to identify the emotional driver and you'll understand your cravings rather than fighting against them.

Alice had been snacking several times a day when she wasn't hungry. She began asking herself, "What do I really want?" She realized that she really wanted a break from her computer. She realized that a better way to give herself a break was to stretch or go for a 10 minute walk. By taking care of the positive need (getting a break) in a positive way, she was able to release 15 pounds in six weeks, just through changing this simple habit.

Our habits can have all sorts of meanings connected to them. Here's just a few my clients have noticed:

Snacking gets me a *break* from my computer

Chocolate means happiness: when I eat chocolate, *I feel happy.*

Eating fast food means I am *independent* and I can do what I want.

Craving sugar cereals means someone is *taking care of me* (like when I was home and my mom would feed me cereal every morning).

Hot fudge sundaes mean I am *connected to my mom.*

Eating sweets gives me *enjoyment.*

Stuffing myself at dinner *reassures me* that I won't go hungry.

Another way to find the meaning or emotional driver is to go through this exercise of filling in the blank. Go through this exercise quickly noticing the first responses that come to mind, these first responses are from your unconscious mind.

I do the habit of _____ so I can feel _____

Go through this exercise several times and notice what responses come to mind. What are the feelings driving the habits and behaviors?

NLP Principle: Underneath all the behaviors that get in our way is an underlying desire for something positive.

Rather than going through the negative behavior to connect with the positive feeling or sense of something, it's even more useful to connect with the positive feeling first. Just like the exercise we did in Chapter One – identifying the higher purpose behind the goal – there is also a higher intention behind the negative behavior that was developed as a way to get something positive.

Identify your top three habits and triggers. Next, identify what you'd rather be doing instead of the old habit and identify a better way to connect with this feeling. Follow these steps below:

Step 1: Identify the habit.

Step 2: Identify the trigger. When do I do this habit?

Step 3: What is it I really want (the feeling or sense of something)?

Step 4: What I would rather do to connect with this feeling?

I often hear that eating sweets is about life enjoyment. If we limit our life enjoyment to food, we not only gain weight, but we miss out on life enjoyment in other ways. We need to open our awareness to enjoying life more and expanding our sense of fulfillment and happiness.

We don't have to enjoy life only through eating pastries or whatever our drug of choice may be. We can enjoy life more by going on walks, reading books, and spending more time doing the things we love. It's almost like we get tunnel vision when food becomes the avenue for connecting with what we desire. As we take off the blinders and pay attention to connecting with what we really want in life, our cravings subside and even disappear.

Identify what the behavior is trying to get for you – and find a new strategy for connecting with the positive feeling. This is the key to changing any habit, craving, or addiction!

Reducing Inner Conflict and Struggle

The NLP parts integration process, which I used with Roger, offers great insight into understanding our motivations and is essential to reducing the struggle and creating internal alignment for moving beyond the old habits. Remember, NLP tools engage as much of the brain as possible, thus the reason for using the hands to represent the habit and the change, engaging pictures, images, and more.

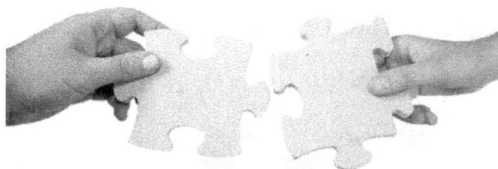

Here are some things to consider before you get started.

Process Notes: When you are creating agreement with the part of you in charge of the old behavior, it's important to give it something else to do instead. This new job or focus should take care of the positive intention behind the behavior. Giving this part a new job can be as *easy as a new mental strategy or thought pattern* rather than a physical task, although Roger's strategy was going to the gym.

Re-sourcing: Re-sourcing (with a hyphen) refers to giving that part of you the resources (the positive thoughts or feelings) that the part is trying to get from the old behavior. For the example below, we'll use Roger's sense of courage. By taking care of the "positive intention" driving the old behavior (desire for courage) and using internal mental strategies to connect with the feeling, the old behavior transforms. By internalizing the positive strategies, there is no need to replace the habit with a new habit. It can all be internal and automatic.

Example of Re-sourcing: Remember, symbols and imagery speak directly to our unconscious mind, which is where cravings and addictions are rooted. From Roger's story, courage came up as the driver behind drinking. As I asked Roger to identify an image or symbol of courage, the image of a lion came to him. He then imagined seeing the image of the lion, shrinking it, and gave it to the part of him in charge of the old behavior *so that it knows it can always be connected with courage,* even as simply as thinking about it!

Note: If you get stuck with this process, I highly recommend working with a qualified Master NLP Practitioner. In the field of NLP, there is a vast background of subtleties in understanding these processes that is difficult to convey in a few pages. A skilled practitioner can help you address the intricacies connected to your original problem.

NLP Tool: Parts Integration (Modified)

Step 1: Set Up. Hold your hands out in front of you as if you are ready to receive a gift with your palms up, your feet flat on the floor, your elbows at right angles, and your hands about 8 inches or so above your knees. If you could package the problem and put it into one hand, notice which hand it seems to fit with best. Let that hand represent the problem. If you find that one hand doesn't connect with the problem more than the other, just imagine packaging it up and choosing a hand to represent it.

Step 2: Compare. Now, turning your attention to the other hand, notice what you experience there at the same time. So, if one hand represents the problem, what does this hand represent? You may notice pictures, images, words, feelings, or sensations.

Step 3: Positive Intention. Turning your attention back to the hand that holds the problem, ask the part in charge of the behavior, "What is this trying to get for me?" (What is the positive intention behind the behavior?) Often the first response that pops into your head is from your unconscious mind, and there may also be more than one answer. Usually the answer is a sense of something. If you get a tangible response, for example, money, ask yourself, "What does that represent for me?"

Ask yourself, "What does that get for me?" a few times to find the intangible sense of something, just as we did in Chapter One when we were looking for the higher purpose of the goal.

Step 4: Redirect. Now ask yourself, "What would be a better way of connecting with that feeling?"

Step 5: New Focus. Now ask the part in charge of the old behavior, "Would it be willing to be in charge of the new focus so that you can better connect to the positive feeling?"

Step 6: Positive Intention. Turning your attention to the other hand, ask that part, "What does it represent? What does it want for me?" If you keep asking the question, you will find that the higher intentions or desires of both hands will eventually match up and sound similar.

Step 7: Acknowledge and Appreciate. Now, turn your attention to the part that holds the problem and ask yourself, "What can this part appreciate about what the other hand is trying to do for me?" Get an answer:

Now, turning your attention back to the other hand, ask yourself, "What can this hand appreciate about what the other hand is trying to do for me?"

Now ask yourself, "How does each part feel now that it is recognized and appreciated?"

Note: Roger replaced drinking with going to the gym. The part of him in charge of drinking agreed to be a motivator and reminder for going to the gym. Give the part a new job or focus and get the agreement. If you are not getting agreement, play with the new job and make sure it fits the positive feeling.

Step 8: Align to Your Outcome. Turn your attention to the positive future you are now creating; see it out in front of you. What does it look like for you? Now ask yourself, "How can both of these parts work together to create that positive future?"

Step 9: Integration. Your conscious job is to be a passive observer. Just notice what comes to mind-thoughts, pictures, images, and so on. Say this phrase out loud: "I ask my *unconscious* mind to begin moving my hands together, but only as quickly as it is able to integrate these parts at all the right levels, all the right ages and places of me, as they are creating harmony and alignment with the positive future I am even now creating."

Again, your conscious job is to be a passive observer. My clients often close their eyes, directing their attention internally.

As your hands are moving together, you might notice resistance, which indicates an objection. If you notice resistance from either hand, address the objection in a positive way until you feel your hands drawing together. Allow your fingers to interlace. Let the movement happen naturally. Typically, the hands will move together slowly and may take as much as 20 minutes. As your hands come together, you should have a positive feeling of well-being.

Step 10: Acknowledge the Integration. Bring your hands to your heart and take a deep breath as you allow these changes to be integrated at all the right places, all the right levels, all the right ages of you. Take all the time you need in the next few seconds and minutes until it feels complete.

This tool is amazingly effective at shifting habits, cravings, and even addictions. Part of the key is that there may be several "parts" associated with a behavior or craving, so you'll want to be thorough or even run through this exercise several times.

Chapter 4:
End Emotional Eating

"I've been eating my emotions!" Jill exclaimed this revelation as we gathered for class. "Anytime I get upset, I've been reaching for food to change how I feel."

If you have been "eating to stuff your emotions" you'll find this chapter useful for beginning to unravel the knots of emotions, feel more neutral, and be more able to choose what you feel.

When I first started working with teen therapy groups, we often started our day by doing a feelings check. Sitting in a circle, each person would say what he or she was feeling that day. I dreaded feelings checks. I never really knew what to say, so I always found the publicly acceptable answer and said something like, "I feel happy" or "I feel hopeful today." These surface answers were safe and not entirely untrue.

After I muddled my way through many feelings checks with lame half-hearted but safe answers, I realized that it was hard for me to identify emotions because I didn't feel just one! I felt a whole bunch of emotions all at the same time and all knotted up together. I felt hopeful and yet disturbed and excited, and even added a side of worry for good measure.

When I learned to identify and be okay with emotions, both mine and others', it became easier. I felt more even tempered, my mood leveled out, and I had a stronger base for feeling neutral. I found I had more choices in how I felt and how I responded.

Strategies

A common strategy for dealing with emotions is to avoid them. We may turn from distraction to distraction. Whether it's food, or alcohol, or movies, or people, these distractions may save us from emotions for awhile, but if we don't take care of them, the emotions get stuffed away and lurk below the surface, festering.

Stuffing our emotions is a way of not dealing with them, it's simply ignoring and denying them. Over time it can lead to a host of problems including increased stress and emotional eating, and it even takes its toll on our physical health. Stuffing emotions gives us less control because they accumulate, eventually leading to an emotional explosion and blowup. Denial is a destructive strategy.

Rather than denying and stuffing emotions, let's try a new approach. Here are some strategies for unraveling the knots of emotions, making sense of what we feel, and putting emotions in proper perspective.

The first step is awareness and acknowledgment. Maybe you've found yourself tied up in knots with emotions. Before we can be aware of our feelings, we have to know it's okay to feel them.

It's okay to feel what you are feeling.

First, give yourself permission to feel what you are feeling. Every emotion has its place. Whatever you are feeling is okay; you are not wrong for what you *feel*. Don't make yourself wrong or others wrong for feeling a feeling. We may have spent a lot of time trying to cover up our emotions; we try to avoid them or distract ourselves from them. But over time ignoring our emotions or covering them up just confuses the issues and then we get knotted up in a ball of emotions.

When you have an emotion, take the time to notice it rather than dismissing it or ignoring it or distracting yourself from it. Ask yourself, "What is this emotion? What am I feeling?" Find words to describe the feeling.

Ask yourself, "What am I feeling?"

Emotions are messengers! They are communicating to us important information about ourselves, our lives, our relationships, and what we like and don't like. Negative emotions point us to what is not working for us. Positive emotions let us know what we like and what is working for us.

So, honor your emotions. Allow yourself to feel what you are feeling – whatever it is – and pay attention to the message. Feelings are important; they help us navigate to a happier life when we notice what's working and change what isn't working.

If you've noticed a difficulty identifying what you feel, you can engage your creative mind to unravel emotions by using this exercise:

Unravel the Ball of Emotions

Step 1: Notice the mass of emotion. Where in your body do you feel it? Now, imagine pulling it out of you and hold it in a ball in front of you. What does it look like? Notice all its colors and identify the colors out loud or write them down.

Step 2: Imagine running your fingers through the mass, untangling the ball as if its pieces of yarn and you are separating the colors. Notice each color, and one by one identify what emotion each color represents. Maybe purple represents calm and red represents passion. There are no wrong answers in how your mind represents color, and the meanings are unique to you. The use of color helps your mind sort through and identify the mixture of emotions.

Step 3: Name each emotion – disappointment, despair, guilt, fear – whatever comes up for you. As you name each emotion you demystify the overwhelming mass, turning it identifiable emotions that you can deal with, and that may be giving you important information about your life.

Step 4: Ask yourself, "What is this emotion telling me?" If it were offering you a message, what message would it be? If there were a positive action the emotion was asking you to take, what would that be?

Emotions may have a few layers connected to them; as you learn to unravel the layers, they become easier to navigate. By going through this process, you will begin to understand the layers of emotions connected to any situation. Try it out now, using either how you feel today or how you felt with a past situation or event.

Identifying what you feel can give you a sense of power through awareness and acknowledgment.

Emotions are messengers. Identify the message of each emotion by asking, "What is this telling me?"

Although emotions are just messengers, unraveling the message can be tricky. Our emotions can range from simple to complex. At the simple level, emotions can indicate something about our environment, such as having a conversation with someone who is condescending. You might notice feeling belittled or small or even angry. The feeling is telling you, "I don't like this."

We can have habits in our emotions, just like the connection with Pavlov and his dogs or my example of chocolate chip cookies, the cookies had the association of being connected to my family. Whatever we repeat over time our brain turns into a habit. The same can be true of our emotions. These "emotional habits" run when triggered by cues, which can include environmental triggers, people, conversations, and so on.

Then, at a deeper level we can have belief patterns underlying our emotions-when our emotions point to underlying thoughts or ideas we have picked up about ourselves or the world around us. In Chapter Five we'll talk more about these patterns and how to change them.

Negative emotions often point to a thought that isn't working for you. If you are experiencing negative emotions such as feeling depressed or angry, look for the thought behind the emotion. By changing the negative thought, you can also change the emotion.

Behind every emotion is a thought.
What thought caused the emotion?

Behind every emotion is a thought. Ask yourself, "What was I thinking that caused this emotion?" If you have a negative emotion, you will find a negative thought behind it. If you wake up, see yourself in the mirror, and begin to criticize yourself for what you are not doing, how do you feel? You would feel down, deflated, and even depressed.

Recognize that emotions are the results of your thoughts and mental habits. What is the thought behind your emotion?

Question the thought and be kind to yourself.

Do you really believe the thought? Does it pass the six-year-old test: If you were to repeat the thought to a room of six-year-olds, would it be appropriate? Would you stand in front of a room of six-year-olds and criticize them for everything they weren't doing right?

Of course not. We recognize that criticizing them would deflate their sense of self and they'd be more withdrawn and less likely to try again.

We often speak to ourselves in ways we wouldn't dream of speaking to others. If it doesn't pass the test, it's not appropriate, so change it. Offer the same compassion and understanding to yourself.

How would you treat a six-year-old who had the negative thought? You would respond with compassion and understanding. So, do the same for yourself. Change the thought and you change the feeling.

If you want to feel better, you need to choose better thoughts.

As adults we may know the "right" things to think and feel, but it's almost as if each of us has an inner six-year-old who didn't get the updates. It's as if this part of us is still operating from the six-year-old mind or is carrying the emotional baggage from a younger frame of reference.

We think, "I know I shouldn't be thinking this," but there is the thought or feeling anyway. Rather than berating, criticizing, and blaming, let's treat ourselves with kindness. You might even imagine that the part of you with the negative thought is a six-year-old child. Ask it, "What do you really want?"

When I work with clients to transform negative self-talk, the part in charge of negative self-talk is usually copying parents or trying to motivate the self to be better. Of course, we respond to negative self-talk the same way we respond to negative communication: we feel down and more withdrawn; we hide who we are and are less motivated.

When that six-year-old part of us recognizes a new strategy to get what we really want – which is usually a feeling – the old behaviors simply disappear in favor of the new strategy. Just like in the exercise in Chapter Three for transforming cravings, you can even use the same process for transforming negative self-talk.

Give yourself what you really want! Once again we come to the underlying desire for a positive feeling. What is this part trying to get for you? What positive feeling do you really want?

You can choose a new feeling by choosing a new thought.

As you acknowledge your emotions and pay attention to the messages, the negative emotion will pass and you can move on to finding a new feeling.

If you want to feel better, you need to choose better thoughts. Reach for a better thought and you will find a better feeling. It can be as simple as giving yourself positive encouragement and support.

What do you like about yourself? What do you like about your life? What is working for you?

Nourish yourself with positive thoughts.

A little game I like to play is, "What would it be like if...."

Whenever you ask a question, your mind has to find the answer. If you ask yourself the right question, you come out with a positive feeling. You can direct the question to find a positive feeling. Ask yourself, "What would it be like if I truly appreciate who I am right now?"

What would it be like if I truly appreciate who I am right now?

Notice how you feel after asking that question and just soak in that feeling. Notice what that is like. You can even imagine carrying the positive feeling into the future, through the rest of today, tomorrow, the next week, the next week, through the next month, three months, six months, and so on as if you are paving your future with this positive feeling – and then bring it back to you in the present moment. This little future preview helps your mind to pave your future with the positive feeling, in a way making it more accessible to you.

I love this tool because the mind and body can respond very quickly.

If you are feeling an extreme emotion, such as anger, reaching for happiness or contentment can be too far to jump. So, choose a more neutral feeling instead:

"I feel angry; what would it be like to just let anger go and feel okay right here, right now?"

Here are some other ways you can use this question.

What it would be like if . . .

I felt okay in my body right here and now?

I felt comfortable with who I am?

I just accept myself as I recognize I am doing the best I can?

Practice making new phrases that point to positive feelings. Positive feelings fuel your motivation and drive.

Be sure you are not just covering up a feeling. Make sure you have gone through the other steps of acknowledging the feeling and paying attention to the message. But when you have the message, you can then move on from the negative emotion. You don't have to stay in it; you can let it pass and then reach for a new feeling.

Sticky Emotions

The difficulty in working with emotions is that some of our thoughts are habits, and they can happen so quickly that we don't even notice them running through our mind.

Sometimes our emotions run wild because they trigger a mental habit or belief such as "I'm not good enough." We then respond and end up with a feeling. Our emotions may also point to beliefs that are not working for us.

If we feel down and we learned to connect food and positive emotions, our unconscious mind will run through the list of foods that mean "feeling better" and may translate one of them into a craving. Of course, this situation can lead to a downward spiral: I'm feeling down so I reach for comfort foods; after I eat them, I feel guilty for eating them so I feel worse so I crave comfort, so I reach for more comfort foods, and on and on.

We can also change this downward spiral to an upward spiral. We now know that we don't need to reach for food to have a positive feeling; we just need to acknowledge how we feel, transform the feeling, and reach for the positive feeling that the food represents.

Jean and Her Mother

It was week four of our healthy lifestyle class. As everyone settled into chairs, I began the group and asked, "Let's check in. How did everyone do this week?"

Jean blurted out, "It was horrible! I ate everything in sight. I couldn't stop myself from eating until I devoured the whole bag of potato chips, a large bag of M&Ms, and anything else I could get my hands on. I just feel awful."

Up until this point, Jean had done really well. We had discussed nutrition and better choices, so it wasn't that she didn't know what foods to choose. She had even noticed the difference that healthy eating made for her health and energy, so I asked, "Jean, what was different this week than the past four weeks?"

Jean said, "Nothing." She paused, then added as an afterthought, "My mom came to visit." The light of awareness spread over her face as the rest of the class giggled with the revelation.

In Jean's experience, her history with her mom led her through a series of mental and emotional habits (already wired into her brain). They happened so quickly that she wasn't aware of the thoughts; she was aware only of the feelings and the compulsion of eating to change the feeling.

Jean explained that her mom was always trying to "fix" her. The message Jean got was that Mom didn't approve of her life, though she was probably only trying to help. That feeling of lack of approval pointed to the underlying idea or belief, "I'm not good enough." Jean felt she wasn't measuring up to Mom's expectations.

So, we see how emotions can get tricky. Jean had her mental triggers tripped when Mom came to visit. Jean felt depressed and so began reaching for foods to feel better. The depressed feeling pointed to an underlying belief or mental habit, "I'm not good enough." In an effort to feel better, the unconscious mind ran through the food lists of which foods meant comfort and approval – M&Ms and potato chips – and the unconscious mind then turned it into a craving or a compulsion to finish the bags.

Let's use the process of unraveling emotions with Jean's example:

In Jean's case, what was Jean feeling? Jean felt belittled, depressed, and even resentment toward her mom; she then felt guilty about feeling resentful.

What was the emotion telling Jean about the situation? That Jean's and Mom's interaction wasn't working.

What was the thought behind the emotion? I must be broken because Mom keeps trying to fix me, or I'm not good enough – as a mental habit or belief. Habits or beliefs often happen so quickly that we are not aware they are firing; we mainly notice the feeling.

What was the emotion telling Jean about herself? That she had an underlying ingrained feeling or belief of not being good enough.

Great! Now we have the core issue, and in Chapter Five we will explore how to change old beliefs – or mental habits and emotional habits. Even if you've carried them around your whole life, you can change them! You don't have to continue to cope or compensate; you can simply replace the old belief by having your brain make a new mental habit.

What positive action was the feeling asking Jean to take? Several actions would be useful: tell Mom how she felt, find her own inner approval for herself, and change the underlying belief.

Note: Taking a positive action is generally easier when the underlying belief has changed because it will drain out the emotional energy attached. When you are able to see the situation from a more balanced or neutral place, positive action is easier to recognize.

The difficulty with our family members is that we are often caught in the old cycles of triggers, negative beliefs, and negative feelings. We can also have communication habits with those close to us when we get caught up in these old cycles. However, when we address the underlying beliefs, we are less likely to be triggered the same way.

Take Responsibility for Your Emotions

Sometimes we blame others for how we feel. We may say, "You make me angry" or even "He makes me happy." When we put other people in charge of our emotions or blame other people for what we feel, we hand over our responsibility and essentially our power.

Rather than making others responsible for what we feel, we must acknowledge that our emotions are okay, our emotions are about us and our relationship to ourselves and our environment.

Your emotions are your own. When you take responsibility for your feelings, you acknowledge your own power. No one else is responsible for what you feel. What is the feeling telling you about yourself, the situation, or the other person? If something isn't working for you, what do you need to change?

If you try to change another person, you will be in for a struggle. You'll find better results in changing your response rather than waiting for the other person to change. When you change your response, you affect the system; very likely the outcome will change too. What can you change within your response?

You are in charge of what you feel. Acknowledge the emotion and pay attention to the message. If it points to a mental habit or belief, you will find the tools for rewiring it in Chapter Five.

You Are Much More than an Emotion

As a child I had extreme emotions, and they were quite bothersome. I would often find myself in the grips of intense disappointment, tantrums, and many tears. I even remembered thinking, "If only God would take away my emotions, then I could be happy." Notice the irony!

Emotions have an interesting place in our world. When we talk about emotions, we often say "I am happy" or "I am sad" as if the definition of who we are is tied up in what we feel. The reality is this: We are not an emotion; we are not a feeling. Emotions are just something we feel.

Change how you express your emotions. Rather than saying "I *am* sad," say instead "I *feel* sad," which helps your mind notice that you are not the feeling. Who you are is greater than any emotion, any event, or any history.

Begin changing how you talk about your emotions and you will find more flexibility in moving out of an emotion.

Notice the internal difference when you say "I *am* depressed" versus "I *feel* depressed." The internal difference is very slight, but if it's just something you feel rather than a definition of you, you can acknowledge the feeling and move beyond it to find a new feeling.

Let's stop defining ourselves by our emotions. Recognize that you are more than an emotion; you are more than any event you have lived. You are more than the sum of your past. You are more than all of it. Emotions are just messengers.

Changing how you express emotions is another way to quickly transform an emotion that feels stuck. Again, pay attention to any messages, mental habits connected, or even beliefs the emotion may be showing you.

NLP: Layers of Emotions

Sometimes when we have an intense emotion we can get stuck, as if it is the only feeling we can have. Emotions can have layers to them. Imagine that the emotion you are feeling is in front of you, and imagine pulling up that emotion and looking under the layer. What's under that emotion? Continue to imagine going underneath each layer, until you reach a neutral state. This will help you transform any negative emotion. Here's an example of how it works:

Ask: What is the emotion I am feeling?

Answer: Anger

Ask: What is under that emotion?

Answer: Hurt

Ask: What is under that emotion?

Answer: Sadness

Ask: What is under that emotion?

Answer: Acceptance or Neutral

Ask: What is under that emotion?

Answer: Stillness

Ask: What is under that emotion?

Answer: Peace

As you pull up the layers, keep asking the same question: What is under that emotion? Sometimes it may feel ominous, like it's a black hole or vast nothingness. It may seem scary at first, but recognize it's just a feeling, notice it, imagine going to the middle of it, looking under it; what's under that layer?

Sometimes the neutral state seems like nothing or "I don't know." Treat the nothingness as a layer and look underneath it. As you drop through the layers of emotion you'll find more neutral states, and then you'll find gradually more positive states. Keep going until you at least get a neutral state or positive state.

Many of our emotions come from our social interactions, and so having positive communication patterns are important to our emotional health and well-being. Most of us inherited our parents' dysfunctional communication-they just passed on what they knew from their parents.

Most of the arguments we experience are just miscommunication. If you've found it difficult to express what you feel or even if you think your communication is pretty good, try out the following positive communication pattern and see how it works for you. This pattern can help clear up negative communication patterns and misunderstandings.

Positive Communication Pattern

Many of us were never taught to deal with and communicate our emotions effectively. When I worked with teen therapy groups, I taught my students a very effective pattern for talking about what they feel. This is a great communication tool.

There are four parts: *when you, I think, I feel, I need.*

When you: Identify the action or behavior of the other person. Let her know specifically what she is doing that isn't working for you. Make it about the behavior, not the person.

Notice the difference: "When you are a slob" versus "When you leave your socks on the floor." The first sentence makes it personal and insulting; the second is simply about the behavior.

I think: It's not just about what is happening; it's our interpretation of the event, the story in our head that leads to the feeling. When the other person does the action, what do you think it means? What is your interpretation or the story you have about it?

"When you leave your socks on the floor, I think you do it because you know I have to pick them up."

I feel: Identify what you are feeling.

"I feel frustrated; it makes more work for me to do."

I need: Get specific about what you want from the other person. Again, it is about changing the behavior, not the person. Also, don't make it about what not to do, but give clear directions about what to do instead.

What not to do: Don't leave your socks on the floor.

What to do: I need you to put your dirty socks in the laundry.

Remember how I said that the unconscious mind translates words into mental pictures that speak more directly to our unconscious mind? Here is another example of making your words and mental pictures work for you. In giving other people directions, use positive words that translate into clear mental pictures for what you want them to do rather than what you don't want them to do. This works great with kids too!

When you _____

I think _____

I feel _____

I need _____

Let's use this communication pattern with Jean's example. If Jean were to use this with her mother, she might say:

"When you criticize me for my clothes (behavior), I think you don't approve of my life and choices (the interpretation or the story). I feel hurt and belittled (the feeling). What I need from you is to stop criticizing me for the choices I make and offer positive encouragement instead."

This simple communication pattern will help to make your communications more clear and allow for better understanding and support in your relationships. This pattern is great for communicating feelings, but it may not change the relationship overnight.

If we are waiting for the other person to change in order to feel better, you may be waiting a long time. It's much easier to make the change within yourself than it is to change others.

**If your happiness relies on other people,
then you do have a problem.**

As you recognize what your feelings are telling you and you identify the habits and mental patterns they point to, you will be better able to take charge of your emotional atmosphere. You can change your thoughts and pick better feelings. You can connect with an internal feeling of being whole and complete, which allows you to be happier and more centered in your life.

Jean could work on a few levels with this communication. She could work on the relationship with her mom and being clear about the messages she got from her mom.

More important, Jean could work on the relationship with herself. By resolving and changing the underlying belief or program of "I'm not good enough," she can feel more confident with herself and be more self-approving.

Unraveling Emotions

There are many good resources available on emotional intelligence and getting more comfortable with your emotions. The following exercise will give you a good start in allowing yourself to feel your emotions, notice the message, notice the thought, and then reach for a new feeling. You can take charge of your emotions. And when you recognize them for the positive insight they bring, you can make the adjustments to being the happier, more whole, and more complete self that loves your life.

Unraveling Emotions Exercise

Step 1: What are you feeling? Unravel the emotions and identify each one.

Step 2: Acknowledge and feel each emotion.

Step 3: Pick one emotion to focus on and ask yourself, "What is this feeling telling me?"

Step 4: What is the thought that caused the feeling? What do you need to change? Is this feeling a simple habit like an association, is it telling you to take action about your situation, or is it telling you to change how you are thinking?

Step 5: Nourish yourself with positive thoughts.

Step 6: Choose a new feeling.

For many of us, it seems as if we are at the mercy of our emotions. But the truth is, when we identify the emotion and identify the message, we don't have to stay stuck in a negative emotion. By choosing a better thought we can feel a better feeling. This isn't to deny what we are feeling but rather to notice and honor the emotion, recognizing its message and then recognizing that we have the freedom to move forward.

Sometimes emotions keep recurring for us because we haven't identified the message. The messenger keeps trying to deliver the message, but if we are ignoring it, it has to come back again and again. This can be true for depression or for any recurring negative emotion. If we keep ignoring it, we are not dealing with it and we keep bottling it up. When we notice it, name it, and notice the message, we can move out of the negative emotion more easily. Our emotions are useful indicators to show us what we can change and adjust to truly create the life we want.

> **Our emotions are useful indicators to show us what we can change and adjust in our life to truly create the life we want.**

Sometimes emotions are habits, old patterns that run over and over. We can create new patterns for our brain to help us get out of emotions we tend to get stuck in and move forward to better emotional states.

NLP Tool: Chaining States for Changing Emotional Habits

As we create a series of steps, we can help the brain set up a new pathway of learning. Then, through repetition of the process, we can help the brain turn the new pathway into a habit.

Step 1: Line out four or more places on the floor as visual steps to walk through. Identify the negative emotion that recurs or the negative emotion that you tend to get stuck in.

Step 2: What emotion would you like to end up with instead?

Step 3: Because jumping from anger to happy is too far a leap, pick neutral states to go between the negative emotion and the positive emotion.

Step 4: Show these emotions on the floor in order. I like to use index cards with word cues on them, which also gives a visual for your brain to remember.

Step 5: Pair each step with cues using visual reminders, hearing or word reminders, and feeling reminders (visual, auditory, and kinesthetic) to engage the different places of the brain. You can choose colors to pair with each state, words you'd be saying to yourself, and the feeling of each state.

Step 6: Run through the sequence of steps and notice if there are any other steps you need to add to create a flow between the steps. The example below could easily be expanded to include more neutral steps, but for simplicity's sake, I'm using the four depicted below.

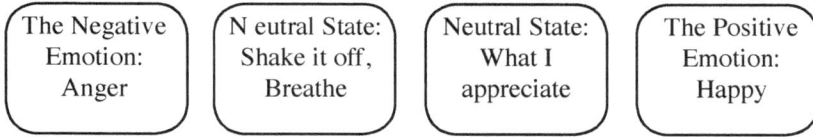

The Negative Emotion: Anger	N eutral State: Shake it off, Breathe	Neutral State: What I appreciate	The Positive Emotion: Happy

Step 7: Run through the sequence; at the end of the sequence look around the room to shift your focus, which tells the brain that the sequence is done.

Step 8: Repeat the sequence five to eight times with a break state (look around the room) at the end of each sequence. The sequence sets up a new mental habit so that when the old emotion is triggered, the brain remembers and has a new way of handling it.

Once again, repetition is key to setting up a new habit. When your brain learns the sequence and you use repetition, you can quickly set up a new emotional habit.

Most of us feel tossed around by our emotions, at the mercy of whichever emotion takes hold of us. We've learned coping strategies to cover up the unpleasant emotions. We eat to distract ourselves; we eat to avoid or deny them. But unless we address the underlying causes-the thoughts that are triggering them-we will continue to feel the emotional pain. There aren't enough doughnuts in the world to fill the space of lonely.

Rather than running from emotions or trying to cover them up or deny them, you'll find a greater ease in navigating emotions as you simply pay attention to them, acknowledge them and then move forward.

As you continue to work with noticing and identifying your emotions and paying attention to the messages they are bringing you, you'll find it easier and easier to release the negatives. You'll find more emotional freedom and even be able to choose how you'd like to feel.

Note: An interesting note regarding how our brain works: We have better access to the memories that reflect our current emotional state. If I feel depressed, my brain accesses memories of times I was depressed. I feel depressed so I think depressing thoughts so I feel depressed, which of course reinforces the depression-creating a vicious cycle of emotion.

By using the Chaining States pattern, you can help your brain break free of the negative cycle and set up better ways to move out of the negative emotions that get in your way.

Family Relationships

As you pay attention to your emotional states, you will pay more attention to how you react with your partner and family. Our communication patterns and our relationship habits can be complicated. If you notice difficulty in this area, you may benefit from working with a good family therapist or relationship coach. Working with professionals can help you and your family members recognize the patterns in your relationships and better see the emotional habits and even the underlying thoughts and beliefs connected to those habits.

One of my clients recognized that she often felt criticized by her husband. It made her feel down and she then felt a need for comfort foods. Reaching for comfort foods fueled the cycle of snacking, gaining weight, and criticizing herself, which, in turn, attracted criticism from her partner. She recognized that the extra weight was, in a sense, insulating herself from her partner. It was protecting her from being vulnerable, even though she wanted closeness and intimacy.

A good family therapist or relationship coach can help you identify these habits and patterns and the collusion between partners in these cycles. Both partners play a role in the relationship dance, and sometimes it's hard to see the part we play on our own. Working with a professional can help you establish better emotional boundaries, build your communication skills, help you see your contribution, and take responsibility so you can improve the situation. If you are struggling in your relationship, with some help you can find better roles to play that are more supportive and enjoyable both for you and your partner.

Often in these roles we play, our partner simply reflects back to us the beliefs we hold about ourselves. Beliefs are ideas that are responsible for our life patterns because they direct what our mind sees. If the beliefs we hold about ourselves are negative, it is likely our relationship will reflect the negative. If the beliefs we hold about ourselves are positive, it is likely our relationships will be positive as well.

When we change the underlying beliefs, those negative thoughts we picked up about ourselves, the patterns often change because what our mind focuses on changes as well. Beliefs are responsible for the patterns that operate our lives. Now let's dive into how the deeper programs of our mind affect these patterns.

Chapter 5:
Our Layers of Awareness

In Chapter One I talked about an image of the iceberg as it relates to how our mind works. Our conscious awareness is the daily action-planning, goal-setting mind and is just the tip of the iceberg. Just below the surface is the subconscious mind, which holds information we use often or have used recently. Below that is our unconscious mind, which holds all our past memories, beliefs, and programs.

Even though we may not consciously remember a past event, like our fifth birthday, it's still recorded in the grand archives of the unconscious mind. For efficiency, our brain stacks memories one on top of the other, with the older memories at the bottom of the pile and the more recent events closer to the top and easier to remember. We don't need to remember the older memories daily; we just need the information we use often or recently.

At the unconscious level, our entire history is stored in our mind along with all the meanings and ideas we've attached to that history. How we experience life is determined by those ideas, which often are perceived as the rules of life and can become the filters of our mind. These filters affect how we see the world and the daily choices we make.

And so we often feel like we are fighting ourselves. Consciously, I know I want to lose weight and I know what I need to do, but if at the unconscious level I have a program to keep a certain weight, I will struggle with visions of doughnuts or whatever your favorite distraction of choice.

We acknowledge such a program mostly as a feeling. It feels like there is a part of us that wants to lose weight and a part of us that doesn't, and this internal struggle is responsible for cravings, lack of motivation, and self-sabotage. We can even feel compelled to do something we know isn't good for us or is unhealthy for us. If we try to suppress the feeling, avoid it, or ignore it, it will surface over and over again. We will continue to struggle unless we transform it at the appropriate level.

Identifying and changing these old programs will finally let you break free of the old cycles of struggle. When these programs are changed, your body weight can normalize naturally and automatically.

We have all been programmed through our history and experiences. The question is: are your programs working for you or against you?

Unconscious Programs: Filters of the Mind

Two people can experience the same event and have very different perspectives. It's not just that we experience an event; it's how we *interpret* the event at the time that makes the difference. These events and the interpretations we've attached to them create beliefs. Beliefs are responsible for how we see and experience the world and are the programs that are operating in our unconscious mind. They are the "tapes" that are playing in our head that motivate our actions.

Beliefs refer to the ideas of who we are and how the world works. As we grew up, we learned many ideas or beliefs to explain life and who we are in it. As children we weren't very well equipped to interpret our experiences and the world around us; however, the ideas we internalized became our beliefs. When these beliefs became habits (wired into the pathways of the brain), they became the programs of our unconscious mind.

These unconscious programs are in our deeper awareness; although we may not be aware of them at the conscious level, they can be very compelling and can even control our experiences. Look at your life. When you identify a pattern that occurs over and over again, chances are there is a belief or unconscious program responsible for it.

An example of an unconscious program comes from one of my colleagues who had been overweight for most of his life. It seemed that his efforts to lose weight just didn't work. Then he began working with the tools of NLP and identified the deeper reasons.

Asking his unconscious mind where this pattern began, he remembered that when he was nine he was bullied by some older kids in the neighborhood. At the time he thought, "If only I were bigger, they couldn't push me around." In his nine-year-old mind, the idea made sense and turned into a belief. Of course he couldn't grow taller, so he grew wider. His unconscious mind ran the program for gaining weight so he could be bigger and stand up for himself.

When he addressed this deeper belief, his weight loss efforts became easier; it was as if the weight simply dropped off, allowing him to slim down to his ideal weight. Weight for him now is no longer an issue. He easily maintains a healthy weight without dieting or struggling.

"It wasn't until I resolved the safety issue that I was able to look at my previous photos and really see just how heavy I'd been. Until then, I hadn't seen myself as overweight. The evidence was there-larger clothes-but when I looked in the mirror, I saw a 'normal size' me. It was like the reverse of anorexia; my mind hid from me that I was overweight until I resolved the old program that was trying to keep me safe." -Rich, Vancouver, WA.

You can see how complex some of these beliefs and issues can be when they operate at the unconscious level. These beliefs even act like filters, so that what we see is a reflection of the underlying belief that reinforces the original belief. In fact, this is a well- known phenomenon in psychology: we will distort, deny, or delete the information that doesn't support our beliefs, thus protecting our perceptions, however untrue.

Body Dysmorphia Disorder

People with body dysmorphia disorder actually see a distorted image of the self. When they look in the mirror their minds distort the image, so what they see is different from reality.

Especially in cases of anorexia, these people see themselves as fat no matter how much they weigh.

If you focus only on their behavior, making them eat, it will be a struggle. Anorexia and bulimia are basically compulsions based on false beliefs. The real problem is in the *beliefs and meanings attached* to thinness. It's not really about the behavior of under eating or overeating; it's really about what they think the *behavior will get for them.*

The messages portrayed in fashion magazines are that women who are thin (even unhealthily so) are more valued and idolized. The underlying driver for thinness could be something like, "If only I am thin enough, then I will be loved or valued." If the underlying beliefs aren't addressed and changed, the problem will continue.

These compulsions are driven by beliefs and are so compelling because they are connected to a core need – a need for love, a sense of being valued as a person, a sense of being okay or acceptance. In shifting this perception, we must address both the underlying need – the belief that is driving the behavior-and create new internal strategies for connecting with the core need of being okay, love, peace, and so on.

Because beliefs are rooted in the unconscious mind, they can be very compelling and intense. Because they exist at the unconscious level, they don't necessarily make sense, and using reason and logic won't really change them. Just being aware of these beliefs is not enough to change them, because they are operating automatically.

NLP and hypnosis offer some sophisticated ways of changing the strategies, the beliefs, and the filters that are responsible for the distorted perception of reality.

If you have really struggled with cravings, addictions, lack of motivation, and self-sabotage, if you recognize recurring patterns in your life, chances are there is a belief behind the scenes perpetuating the cycle. When you change the belief, you break free of the old cycle.

Beliefs: The Hidden Drivers Behind Habits, Cravings, and Addictions

For this exercise, think of the unconscious mind as a highly skilled supercomputer. The unconscious mind is very quick at processing information, much quicker than the conscious mind. Because we are looking for the answers held in the unconscious mind, we want to pay attention to the *very first answers that come to mind*. Even if the answers don't make sense or even if you consciously don't believe them, your first response is what your unconscious mind holds in place.

Assessing Beliefs Behind Habits, Cravings, and Addictions

Think of the habits and cravings that are getting in your way. Then, think of the effects of those habits or cravings.

The Problem: Habit or Craving _____

The Effect of the Habit or Craving _____

Now ask yourself the following three times, pausing each time for an answer. Notice your first responses. Our unconscious mind is much quicker at processing information than our conscious mind, so as you pay attention to the very first responses, this will give you what your unconscious mind holds.

This habit or craving means _____

This habit or craving means _____

This habit or craving means _____

Now try this phrase, and once again, notice the very first response that comes to mind.

I need this (problem) in order to _____

I need this (problem) in order to _____

I need this (problem) in order to _____

Recognize that these beliefs are just ideas. We can tell they are not the rules of life because they aren't true for everyone. For some people losing weight can be easy, maintaining their ideal weight is natural, and exercise is fun.

You can also identify beliefs by paying attention to the associations you have with words and meanings around the problem. As you go through the following list, pay attention to the first things that come to mind.

Remember that our unconscious mind is much quicker at processing information than our conscious awareness, so noticing the first responses will tell you what your unconscious mind is holding in place.

Asking yourself the same question three times will also help bring up the layers of these meanings.

Identifying Your Beliefs

Weight Loss is:

1. _____
2. _____
3. _____

Eating Healthy Means:

1. _____
2. _____
3. _____

I have to carry extra because:

1. _____
2. _____
3. _____

I have to carry extra weight so that:

1. _____
2. _____
3. _____

To let go of the weight I would have to.:

1. _____

2. _____

3. _____

Extra weight keeps me from:

1. _____

2. _____

3. _____

Extra weight saves me from:

1. _____

2. _____

3. _____

When I release the weight I will be:

1. _____

2. _____

3. _____

Beliefs often sound like absolutes – like the rules of life or how the world works. One way to soften them is to change how we word them. For example, going from the belief "weight loss is hard" to "weight loss is easy" may be too big a jump; it may sound like we are lying. However, when we add the word can and say "weight loss can be easy," it opens up that possibility.

Rephrasing Beliefs: Change Your Words

Changing your words is a basic level of softening old beliefs. Pay attention to how you talk about the belief. Then, you can change the words you use which then changes how you think and how you feel.

Write your beliefs about weight loss below; underneath each write what you would rather believe. Use words that create the space for the possibility of the new belief. Just by changing how you talk, you can begin to change what you believe.

For example: If my old belief is that weight loss is hard, I can change it to weight loss can be a natural and easy process. The word can opens up possibility.

1. My old Belief: _____

My New Belief: _____

2. My old Belief: _____

My New Belief: _____

3. My old Belief: _____

My New Belief: _____

4. My old Belief: _____

My New Belief: _____

The unconscious beliefs we carry don't necessarily make sense to the conscious adult mind, but they do make sense to the younger part of us that picked them up and internalized them.

As children, we picked up negative beliefs and ideas from our experiences and the world around us. Even with the best parenting, kids can adopt irrational or negative beliefs. As a parent, you can make a difference with your children by explaining things as they happen and offer positive interpretations for what is happening during life changes and transitions.

Beliefs are just ideas, but because we've repeated them or they've been reinforced through time, they are also habits wired into the neural net in our brains. When they've been turned into mental habits and run automatically, they can run unchecked even though we've continued to grow older. Then these beliefs can get stuck. It's almost as if those unconscious programs don't get the updates that life has changed or that we are older and wiser.

Here is another way to identify unconscious beliefs connected to your problem.

Using NLP to Identify Unconscious Beliefs

The following exercise uses hands polarity, the Parts Integration tool explained in Chapter Four, but asks your unconscious mind to identify the beliefs connected to your problem. Your conscious job through this process is to pay attention to what comes to your conscious awareness.

We all have preferences in how we process information. You might find your information coming more quickly through pictures, or if you are more tuned into feelings, you might notice feelings first. Give yourself some quiet space without distraction to go through this process.

Be aware that the answers may not make sense to you, but to the part of your mind that picked them up, they do. Just allow your mind to be open to what comes to your awareness.

Also, be patient. Give yourself time to go through this exercise – at least 20 to 30 minutes. You should find your hand drifting down slowly as your brain accesses the beliefs connected for you.

The language of the unconscious mind uses pictures, images, symbols, and feelings. For some of my clients, their answers come in phrases and words; for others, there may be memories or feelings that come to mind. So pay attention to whatever comes to mind, even if it doesn't make sense.

This is a good exercise to do with a partner who can take notes for you while you stay focused in the process. Or, you can record yourself talking about the things that come to mind as you go through the process and then listen and sort your responses later.

NLP Tool: Hands Polarity for Unconscious Beliefs

Step 1: In a sitting position, hold your hands out in front of you as if you are ready to receive a gift. You'll want your feet flat on the floor and about 6 to 12 inches between your hands and knees.

Step 2: Think of the problem (carrying extra weight) and imagine packaging it up and putting it into one hand or the other. Notice which hand it fits with best.

Step 3: Turning your attention to the other hand, notice what you experience there by contrast at the same time.

Step 4: Turn your attention back to the hand that holds the problem and say, "I ask my unconscious mind to begin lowering my hand, but only as quickly as it is able to bring to my awareness the beliefs that have created this as a problem for me."

Step 5: Your conscious job is to notice anything that comes to mind-images, symbols, pictures, words, phrases, sounds, and feelings.

Write your responses on the left, whatever came to your mind during the process. Then, identify what belief or idea the thought or feeling points to and write that on the right.

The next step is to take your list and notice how you feel about the beliefs or ideas. You may also identify which ones carry more emotional energy with them. By noticing which ones are more emotionally charged, you will identify the stronger beliefs. These will be good ones to start changing first.

Images, Thoughts, Feelings   **The Beliefs**

_____   _____

_____   _____

_____   _____

_____   _____

_____   _____

_____   _____

_____   _____

_____   _____

Here are some of the beliefs I uncovered in working with my clients:

Being healthy means eating as much food as possible.

Carrying extra weight means I'm saving for future times of famine.

If I am bigger, I can stand up for myself.

I am overweight so I can be happy; being thin means being unhappy and high-strung.

I am resentful toward my partner, so I will make myself less attractive to get back at him.

Carrying extra weight protects me from getting close to people.

Next, looking over your list and rate your beliefs. Using a scale of 1 to 10, rate each for how strongly the belief resonates for you. Mark your ratings to the right of The Beliefs. You'll want to change the highest ranking beliefs first.

A belief is simply an idea that has become a mental habit wired into the brain. Beliefs can run automatically as "unconscious programs."

A habit is a pathway of neurons in the brain that fires when triggered. Beliefs are mental habits that run automatically as unconscious programs. Habits and beliefs are responsible for the repeating patterns in life, whether it's struggling with weight over and over, or difficulty with relationships, or even patterns around career or finances. Behind these patterns are beliefs shaping your perspective and perpetuating the cycles, acting as a self-fulfilling prophecy. When we change the beliefs, our life patterns change as well.

Why do we know which foods are bad for us but find ourselves craving them anyway? If I carry the belief (at an unconscious level) that it's better to be heavy, I will find myself eating the wrong foods, snacking at the wrong times, and feeling no motivation for fitness. Or, if I have the belief that losing weight is hard work, I will be attracted only to weight loss programs that are hard. I might find myself really struggling as I exert a lot of effort, which then proves that the belief is correct.

However, when you change the belief, you actually change the rules. Beliefs feel like the rules of life (even if they are irrational), and when you replace the old beliefs with new beliefs, you find your motivation; you can stay focused and achieve your goals.

What would it be like if the following were your beliefs, the foundation for how your mind operates in regard to your health, weight, and wellness?

- It's easy to eat healthy.

- Weight release can be easy and natural.

- I love fitness; it feels good to move my body.

- It's fun and easy to be fit and healthy.

- I enjoy all the health and vitality that fresh foods offer my body.

- I love my body and all that it does for me, and I am committed to taking care of it.

- My body is working for me, naturally maintaining my ideal healthy weight.

When you change your underlying beliefs, you change the filters of how your mind operates. Your beliefs focus your brain and attention to either notice or discredit your experience. If you have negative self beliefs at the unconscious level, you will discredit the compliments that come your way and pay attention to the criticisms instead.

When you change your beliefs, you open up a whole new experience of life, because you tune your brain to a different experience. It's a little like wearing glasses: how we see the world and our experience of it has everything to do with the filters of our mind-the glasses we wear. If you don't like how the world looks, change the glasses you are wearing by changing your beliefs. Use the space below to change your glasses.

Identify the negative beliefs and list them in the column on the left. Then, identify the opposite belief or the antidote and list them on the right.

Change Beliefs

Your Old Belief

Opposite Belief/

It's hard to lose weight

It's easy to lose weight

_____ _____

_____ _____

_____ _____

_____ _____

_____ _____

_____ _____

_____ _____

Consciously, beliefs may not make sense, but they can still carry strong feelings. It's why affirmations are only partially effective; they don't address the underlying feelings and mental habits, and they don't feel real.

Affirmations are simply positive statements. As you say these positive statements to yourself, you notice that you feel good. Once again, it's our thoughts that create our feelings. The problem with affirmations is that they feel good for the moment we think about them, but then we forget and slip back into our everyday mental patterns.

However, by using an NLP approach, we can boost the effectiveness of affirmations and begin changing the mental habits that get in the way.

Good affirmations are written in the present tense, they are stated in the positive, and they inspire positive feelings. Write your affirmations about how you would like to be or what you would like to experience.

Here are some positive affirmations that will be useful for you in the weight loss journey. If the "I am" statements don't feel real, insert the word can.

- I accept myself as I
  am right now.

- I appreciate my body and all that it does for me.

- I can love my body and appreciate who I am now.

- I am easily releasing the excess weight.

- I take care of myself and put myself first.

- I am slimming down naturally to my ideal healthy weight.

- Making healthy choices is easy for me.

- I enjoy healthy foods.

- I enjoy (can enjoy) fresh fruits and vegetables.

- My body is comfortable.

- It feels good to be me.

More than Affirmations

Start with an affirmation, then make it more effective by incorporating more places of the brain: use visual (what you see), auditory (what you hear), and kinesthetic (what you feel) cues to activate more places of the brain, thus creating a better reminder system.

Affirmation: I am a happy and healthy person.

What do you see? I see yellow sunshine over my head.

What do you hear? I hear laughter.

What do you feel? I feel laughter in my chest and a smile on my face.

Affirmation:

What do you see?

What do you hear?

What do you feel?

Affirmation:

What do you see?

What do you hear?

What do you feel?

Affirmation:

What do you see?

What do you hear?

What do you feel?

Affirmations are one way to start addressing old beliefs, but they are more like a band-aid approach. Part of the reason affirmations don't stick is that they are not integrated to the chain of neurons firing during an old belief. Remember, a mental habit is a chain of neurons firing together, a default pathway in the brain.

An even more effective way to change old beliefs is by engaging the old pathway and creating a new chain of steps so that when the old pathway is triggered, the brain will fire the new chain of steps and end up with a new belief or the positive affirmation.

Rather than taking a lot of conscious energy and focus in repeating an affirmation, we can actually help the brain set up a new pathway and use repetition to turn it into a habit. When it becomes automatic, your brain will be working for you!

Change a Belief by the Chaining States Process

When you've identified the belief you want to work with, line out a series of steps on the floor. With NLP processes, physically walking through these steps helps your brain set up and link together the new pattern of thinking while engaging your body's nervous system. And, by using repetition you can create a new habit around your old belief.

This process is based on the NLP Chaining States process. By creating a sequence of states or stages and then walking through it repeatedly, your mind will turn the sequence into a habit.

NLP Chaining States

By lining out these spaces on the floor and physically walking through this process (rather than just thinking about it), it engages more of the processing centers of the brain. This helps set up the new sequence as a new habit more quickly. By physically walking through each step, your body will create a new habit in your neurology as well.

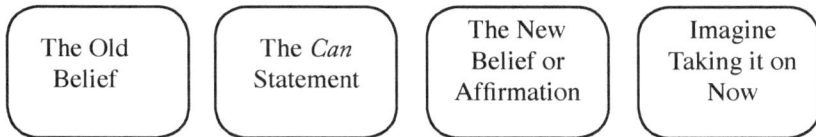

The Old Belief	The *Can* Statement	The New Belief or Affirmation	Imagine Taking it on Now

Step 1: Using index cards or paper squares, on the floor line out the steps in sequence as shown in the diagram.

Step 2: Stand in the first square and say the old belief; notice how the old belief makes you feel. Example: It's hard to lose weight.

Step 3: Take a step into the next square and say the Can statement. Example: Weight loss can be natural.

Step 4: Step into the next space and say the new belief you'd rather be living by. Example: Weight loss is natural and easy.

Step 5: Imagine you are living the new belief now. What would you be seeing? What would you be thinking or saying to yourself? How would it feel?

Step 6: Walk around the room saying the new belief out loud, which engages the speaking and hearing centers of the brain. You can engage the sensory and motor centers of the brain by walking and using your hands to emphasize your words, as if you are talking with your hands. By looking around the room, you engage the visual centers of the brain in processing as well.

Step 7: Break the state. Think of something unrelated, like the weather, which tells the brain the sequence is done.

Step 8: Walk back to the first square and repeat this process six to seven times, walking through the sequence with the break state (Step 7) at the end. Repetition will turn the new phrase into a new mental habit.

Check your results: You can tell if you have changed a belief by how you feel when you say the old belief. Say the old belief. Using a scale of 1-10, with 1 being not true and 10 being true, how true does this phrase feel to you now? Compare the two beliefs. Which feels more true for you? As you repeat the steps a few times it will strengthen the positive belief and continue to weaken the old negative belief.

Identity Level Beliefs

In the last section, we looked at beliefs and how they can direct our lives at the unconscious level. Sometimes these beliefs are wired into our identity and they can become a definition of who we are. If we don't replace these definitions, it can be very difficult to stay on track because our unconscious mind holds onto the definition of who we are as the heavier self.

One lady told me, "I lost 60 pounds and did very well for about six months, but every time I saw myself in the mirror, I saw the old me. I never felt like the skinnier person. The weight all came back within the year."

If we aren't integrating *who we will become* as the lighter body, we will continue to struggle. To address this important concept, we must look at the underlying definitions of who we are, the beliefs we hold about ourselves.

"I am" beliefs can be deeply ingrained because they are intertwined with the sense of who we are. These identify beliefs can affect every area of life. One of the most common beliefs I've run across is: I am not good enough.

If this is your definition, your unconscious mind is wired into that perspective, and you notice or pay attention to the ways you seemingly don't measure up and so it reinforces the belief.

Beliefs – and especially beliefs about who we are – act like self-fulfilling prophecies. For example, if your unconscious mind holds the belief "I'm not good enough," you may feel self-conscious in meeting new people and so it's harder for you to meet new people because you feel self-conscious. When you feel self-conscious, you shrink back and are withdrawn and so you don't meet new people. Your mind then interprets the situation as, "see, people aren't interested in me because I'm not good enough."

We can have beliefs attached to the actual habit or to the outcome. They can be unique to each person and they are the underlying reasons the extra weight persists despite our best efforts. These beliefs don't necessarily make sense, but the unconscious mind can continue to perpetuate them even if they are outdated.

Here are some "I am" beliefs my clients have uncovered:

Cleaning my plate means I am a good girl. (belief about a habit)

I am overweight so I won't be as attractive. (belief about an effect)

I am more loveable by being overweight.

I am being nice to other women by being heavy and less attractive.

I am the heavy one in my family.

I don't deserve to be really healthy and enjoy my body.

I am heavy so that I am different – not like the skinny person I know and don't like.

My whole family is overweight. If I were to lose weight, I wouldn't fit in with my family.

The first part of changing these old beliefs is, of course, awareness. Many times they feel like truth, so we are not aware they are with us. As we identify and change these old beliefs, we become better able to create new definitions of who we are that better support us in being the person we want to be.

Your "I Am" Beliefs

What are the beliefs about weight, health, fitness, or habits that are connected with your identity? A good way to identify these beliefs is to ask yourself, "Who am I at my current weight?" and notice what comes to mind.

Another way to identify these old beliefs is to take a look at the beliefs list you identified earlier, and look for recurring themes. Or you can ask yourself, "What does it mean about me that I am overweight or doing the old eating habits?" Notice what comes to mind.

When you identify your core beliefs that are negative, be aware they can feel pretty awful. Remember that these are only ideas and you can choose new ideas, new definitions of who you are. You get to choose what you believe about you. So, be compassionate with yourself. You might even imagine stepping back from the old ideas and looking at them as an observer.

Once again, these beliefs may not make sense to your conscious mind, but they made sense to the younger you who picked them up at an earlier time.

New Beliefs: To begin shifting these beliefs, let's define some new beliefs about who you are as the lighter self or ideal weight, and who you are becoming. Write out some positive I am statements.

You can use the same process of Chaining States for changing these beliefs. Since beliefs were formed from experiences and the mind stores experiences as memories, you may have to overwrite some old memories. One of the easiest ways to do this is to use Eye Circles.

The basis for this exercise is that our eyes hold visual memories. By making circles with our eyes while saying the old belief, our eyes access the old memories associated with the old belief so that we are better able to replace the old wiring with the new belief, essentially overwriting the old files.

This is quite an interesting phenomenon. Try it out: Have a friend sit across from you and ask him to follow your finger as you trace it across his line of vision from right to left and back again. You will notice there are places where the eyes skip or glitches in the eye-tracking patterns. These glitches are related to stored visual memories that our mind tries to avoid and so our eyes skip over these places in the visual field.

Using Eye Circles is a simple way for the eyes to begin overwriting old *visual* memories so the new beliefs are better absorbed and integrated. Using the same process as Chaining States, add Eye Circles before going through the sequence (see the diagram below).

Eye Circles

Step 1: Holding your arm out in front of you with your thumb up, begin by making a sideways figure eight, following it with your eyes and saying the old belief three times.

Step 2: While keeping your head straight, continue to move your thumb in a sideways figure-eight pattern, following your thumb with your eyes and repeating the old belief, saying it out loud a few more times as your eyes move through the pattern. You can also add big circles to the right, then switch direction and do big circles to the left.

Step 3: Then, imagine focusing the old belief onto the tip of your thumb and then throwing it out into space and exploding into a million pieces.

Step 4: Step forward, saying the Can phrase, and then follow the steps through the rest of the sequence.

Note: You'll get better results by physically walking through this exercise rather than just thinking about it.

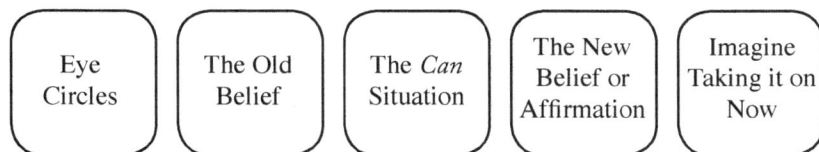

Eye Circles	The Old Belief	The *Can* Situation	The New Belief or Affirmation	Imagine Taking it on Now

It can be tricky to identify the beliefs we hold at the unconscious level, especially when we've learned the more appropriate things to think. Even though we don't consciously believe it, a deeper part of our mind can still hold the old belief or idea. Pay attention to the emotional energy attached to the idea.

A way to test for this is to say the old idea and pay attention to how you feel. You may notice tension in your body when you say the old belief, which is a good indicator that the unconscious mind is running the belief as an old program.

Your Dreams Are Windows

Our dreams are windows to what we hold in the unconscious mind. The unconscious mind is extremely important to how we operate daily. The difficulty is that most of this information is outside our regular awareness. Our unconscious mind speaks through the language of symbols, imagery, metaphor, and feelings more than words.

Some of what we dream about is simply our mind processing our day. However, the dreams which have messages or important information from the unconscious carry a *feeling*, and especially the dreams that carry a *strong feeling*.

Your dreams are a window to the patterns your unconscious mind holds. The messages are not always obvious, so it may take a little bit of interpretation. Dream interpretation books are just those authors' interpretations of symbols and imagery. They don't know how your dream makes you feel or the context of the images within your dream; they don't know what these symbols mean to you. You are the only one who really holds the answers to these meanings because you are the only one who knows what feelings were involved.

Here is one example of a dream I had and my interpretation:

I was at a beautiful wedding and rather than a wedding cake, there were all sorts of specialty cheesecake slices. The wedding had several floors to it, and I kept going from floor to floor, looking for the cheesecake slices, but every time I got to a plate that held the cheesecakes, they were all gone.

Here is how I interpreted this dream. Pay attention to the *themes and feelings*.

What were the *feelings* in this dream? Frustration-there wasn't any left for me.

What was the *context* of the dream? Wedding

What did this context represent to me? Romantic love and relationship

My interpretation: In searching for love and relationship, I was frustrated because my unconscious mind was holding onto the feeling, "There isn't someone for me."

My *feeling* simply pointed to an old belief, and now I could change it!

After I changed this belief and feeling, a significant relationship showed up!

Exercise: When you wake up in the morning, give yourself five minutes to jot down anything you remember from your dreams. Notice particularly the *feelings* involved. What are the themes, feelings, and context of the dream? From this information, what is the belief held by your unconscious mind?

Some dreams are just junk dreams; they don't really mean anything. However, it's the dreams with emotional content or the dreams that stand out in your mind that will have useful information for you.

Before you go to sleep at night, give your unconscious mind direction by simply saying, "I ask my unconscious mind to find and identify for me any beliefs that are getting in the way of my ideal healthy weight." Then, in the morning write down your dreams and go through the interpretation process below.

When you have identified the old beliefs, go through the belief change process and your mind will begin to wire in a new belief and you can upgrade your unconscious programs.

Dream Interpretation

What was the story?

What were the feelings and themes?

What was the context and what does it represent to you?

Put it all together for the interpretation:

Just by asking yourself a few simple questions you can interpret the beliefs that are held in your deeper mind. As you update these old beliefs, you'll discover a freedom to live life on your own terms rather than be destined to repeat the same old patterns over and over.

If you've found your life repeating patterns, chances are there are unconscious programs operating at the deeper level. Breaking free of these old ideas and programs allows you to upgrade your unconscious programs and live your life by your own definitions.

When we truly believe in ourselves, in who we are and what we are capable of, we expand our possibilities for our lives, our health and our happiness. What we thought wasn't possible now opens to us; we can craft our lives by our deepest values and live as the best expression of who we really are.

Weight as A Message from the Unconscious Mind

For many who struggle with extra weight, the weight is only a symptom pointing to a deeper issue. Releasing extra weight is about releasing the fears, the old ideas and limitations, the past baggage, and the negative feelings that have weighed you down and held you back. And as you identify old ideas that aren't working for you and incorporate more supportive beliefs about life and yourself, the old frustrations dissolve and your body can finally normalize.

Here's another way to identify what carrying extra weight represents for you and the unconscious reasons you may be holding. By using imagery and engaging your creative and unconscious mind, you'll quickly identify what the extra weight represents. Here's how this process worked for me.

I had worked for many years as a wilderness guide and back-packer and so keeping in shape wasn't a problem for me. Then I went back to school and my life changed. I was spending my time in classrooms and reading books. I also wasn't taking the time to cook, and I often chose quick and convenient foods.

As I went through the What Weight Represents process that follows, I "packaged up" the 30 pounds I had gained from this lifestyle and set it out across from me. As I shifted to the position of the 30 pounds looking back at me, it dawned on me: I had been eating for adventure. The extra fat represented wanting adventure!

Adventure and freedom had been an important part of my life, and in the past I had found a lifestyle that really expressed those values. I had been working as a backpacker for two weeks out of the month, hiking with teens into the backcountry.

Every week we found ourselves in the wild places, we saw petroglyphs and pictographs and slept out under the stars. We had campfires every night and talked about the meaning of life and what it meant to be human. Every other week, I had a week off, and I would travel and visit family members and friends.

When I went back to school, my life changed. It became very scheduled with classes and textbooks, going to the same places every day and life became very routine. Of course, my lifestyle became more sedentary. Rather than spending time hiking to new places, I spent the bulk of my time reading books and studying.

The inner need for adventure reared its head anytime I saw some new sweet I hadn't tried; it was almost a compulsion. Finding adventure through food, however, isn't a real solution for adventure and it caught up with me.

What I took from the process was the message that I needed to find ways to express freedom and adventure through avenues other than food. I began to give myself time off on weekends to explore local attractions and visit new places. In doing so the compulsion lessened. I could still enjoy foods, but the need to try new sweets subsided.

Rather than berating and criticizing ourselves for the extra weight we've gained, we can recognize that extra weight as a symptom. It can be the result of simple habits, or it can also point to a deeper issue of our unconscious mind. Remember that our unconscious mind speaks to us through feelings, pictures, symbols, and metaphor.

What has been weighing you down? What is the message the extra weight represents for you in finding more fulfillment in the bigger picture of your life?

When we pay attention to the messages our deeper mind is sending us through the body (or through a symptom), we can then address the real issue at the deeper level. We can reduce the internal struggle and allow our mind and body to work together for lasting healthy weight success.

Through the NLP perspective, we see behaviors of the body, even health symptoms, as an expression of the unconscious needs and beliefs. As you increase your self-awareness, you can respond to these patterns rather than fighting them. By addressing the underlying message, you create internal alignment and achieve greater health and well-being naturally.

What Weight Represents Exercise - NLP Perceptual Positions

By shifting your physical positions, you are engaging the brain's spatial orientation as well as creating a "disassociation" with the fat, which helps to access a new perspective. It also helps your unconscious mind work with your creative mind to identify what the fat represents for you.

Line out two spaces on the floor and walk through each step as you shift between the spaces:

```
        ⭕ Self            ⭕ The Fat
```

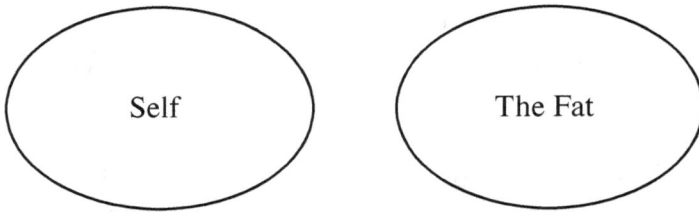

Step 1: Starting in the space of Self, imagine packaging up the extra fat you don't want into a ball; see it out in front of you about 3 or 4 feet.

Step 2: Notice: What do you think and feel about that ball of fat? What does it look like?

Step 3: Walking over to the Fat, imagine stepping into the ball of fat and looking back at yourself. Imagine that the extra weight represents a part of you that wants something. As the fat, what does the fat want? What are you trying to get for the self over there? Notice whatever comes to mind-thoughts, pictures, images, words, or feelings. If there were a positive reason for hanging onto the fat, what would it be?

Step 4: Step back into the Self. Thank the part of you in charge of the fat for its positive reason, and then ask it to transform into its highest positive message for you; imagine surrounding it with light and compassion. As you surround it with light and compassion, watch it transform and notice what new image it turns into now, and what it represents for you now.

Step 5: Ask it to help you transform into your highest potential, and allow the transformed image to come back and integrate with you as the positive changed form as the new image.

Note: This type of exercise draws on your creative and unconscious mind, so if you aren't used to using your creative mind, just give it a little time. Be patient with the exercise and notice any thoughts, feelings, and images that come to mind. Because you may not be used to thinking this way, it may take a bit of reflection to allow the answers to come to mind.

This is a great exercise because it draws on the unconscious mind and can quickly reveal to you what carrying extra weight represents for you. As you pay attention to the message your body is trying to give you through the extra weight, you can more easily release the weight and slim down to your healthy self.

What is the message your mind and body are sending you through the symptom of extra weight? What is the greater message for your life? What actions can you take that will help you address the message in better ways?

Rather than fighting the cravings, struggling against ourselves, and creating a war with our bodies, we can transform the struggle with awareness. Our unconscious mind uses weight as a way of getting our attention. Weight is only a symptom of a deeper issue. But it is just this deeper issue that is the doorway to moving your life forward and becoming your lighter, happier, and more balanced self.

By using awareness, we can appreciate the positive message. By using appreciation and compassion, we can transform the struggle.

NLP Principle: Every part of us is trying to get something positive, even if the behavior is misdirected.

By using awareness, appreciation, and love, we can more quickly transform the problems in our lives into stepping stones. Whether the problem is body weight, a habit, a craving, or emotional reactions to the people around us, self awareness will give you the keys to opening the door for you to what you really want and moving forward.

Rather than fighting and struggling with the problem, you can recognize that in the past many of the problems you worked through held deep answers to learning and growing. As you recognized the problems you overcame in the past, you can also recognize that in overcoming them, you became more capable and more able to move your life forward in some way.

Transform your problems into stepping stones with self awareness and compassion.

In fact, you can even appreciate those problems as avenues of expanding who you are. Every problem in life is an opportunity for learning and growing in a positive way.

Self awareness has the power to heal and transform, whether with ourselves, our bodies, our habits, or even with the people around us. By adopting a higher perspective of compassion and acceptance, we can see through our problems and turn them into stepping stones.

Chapter Six:
The Bigger Picture of Your Life

The reasons for gaining weight or the difficulty maintaining a healthy weight relate to the bigger picture of our lives as we saw with the exercise, What Weight Represents. The Life Balance Wheel from the world of coaching illustrates how all the pieces of our life work together. In the Life Balance Wheel, I place you at the center to represent how life works.

Life Balance Wheel

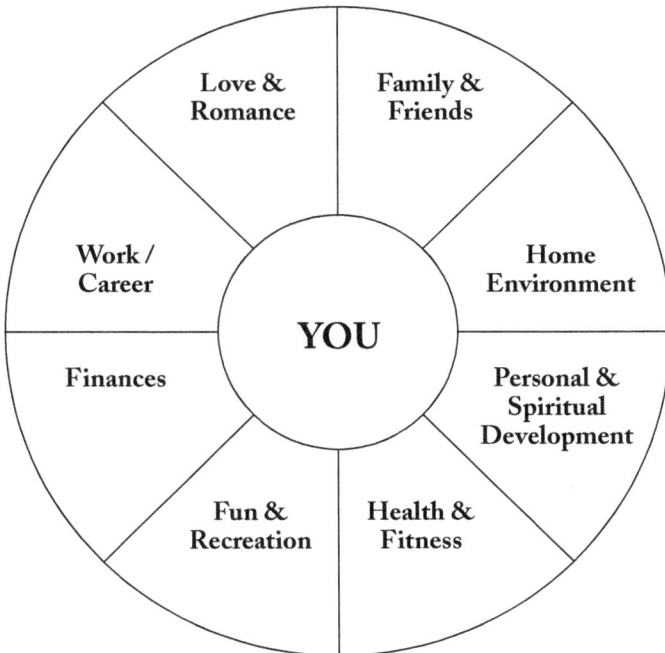

Life Balance Wheel diagram with YOU at the center, surrounded by: Love & Romance, Family & Friends, Home Environment, Personal & Spiritual Development, Health & Fitness, Fun & Recreation, Finances, Work / Career

Your mental and emotional habits and beliefs are central to how your life operates and to your experience of life.

There are many ways to use this tool. One way is to look at your overall life balance. You can also use it to see the flow of health through your life. As you use the wheel, you may also identify themes or patterns that run through several areas of your life.

Life Balance Wheel Assessment

I hear it over and over again: overeating or eating sugar and junk food represents life enjoyment and happiness. If we are escaping to food to find happiness, we are not really living, and our happiness lasts only as long as the ice cream, cookie, or other food distraction we've chosen. Besides, how often do you find yourself indulging in food only to find that you hardly tasted it?

If you are not feeling balanced or *fulfilled* in some aspect of life, you may be using food as a cover-up or an escape. When your mindset becomes balanced, fulfilled, and hopeful, your life can take priority and food can take a backseat, thereby having a more natural fit in your life. We still want to enjoy food, but we want to expand our life enjoyment more! If food has become an escape or distraction from unsatisfied feelings, it's a little like living with blinders on – we begin to focus more and more on food and less and less on the richness and vastness of life.

Try this assessment to see how balanced your life is and to begin to identify what you'd like to change.

Step 1: Using the Life Balance Wheel, on a scale of 1 to 10 rate each area of your life with how satisfied you are (1 being not satisfied and 10 being very satisfied).

Step 2: Color each segment of the wheel according to the rating you gave it. For example, if you rated love and romance a 5, fill it in 50 percent; if you rated fun and recreation a 3, fill it in 30 percent.

Now look at your life wheel. I like this visual of how life is rolling along. How balanced is it? If the wheel was rolling, would it be a bumpy ride or fairly smooth? You may see some areas that are very satisfying and others that need your attention.

Step 3: What changes would you like to make? What would make each area a 10? You can use the left column to prioritize which areas are most important for you to focus on first.

Priority	Area of Life	What would make it a 10 for you?
	Family & Friends	
	Home Environment	
	Personal & Spiritual Development	
	Health & Fitness	
	Fun & Recreation	
	Finances	
	Work & Career	
	Love & Roamnce	

Step 4: Now that you've rated each area, ask yourself, "what would make each area a 10?" These are the positive results that you'd like to see for each area. You can then identify specific goals and actions that you can take to expand your life satisfaction within each area of the life wheel. Prioritize your goals and actions and only take on 2 or 3 new actions each week.

Flow of Health Through Your Life

You can also use the Life Balance Wheel to understand what is working against your health and how to make areas of your life more supportive of better health choices.

Step 1: Identify what is working against your health choices in each area of your life.

Step 2: What is your solution for each area?

Here's an example: You might be aware of a habit of reaching for high-sugar foods in the afternoon, which then causes a crash right after work. Finding that you have little energy and no motivation, you may skip your workout, feel guilty about it, and go home to find you are snippy with your partner because you have low energy.

By going through the Life Balance Wheel, you'll begin to see where these patterns interrelate. As you identify the patterns, even with simple changes you can shift the flow of health through your life.

Now fill in the areas below:

Area of Life	Step 1: What is working against your health choices?	Step 2: What you can do to change it.
Family & Friends		
Home Environment		
Personal & Spiritual Development		
Health & Fitness		
Fun & Recreation		
Finances		
Work & Career		
Love & Roamnce		

Who You Think You Are Runs Your Life

Notice that YOU is at the center of the wheel. You are central to how your life is working. When you add the awareness of your habits (mental and emotional) and your unconscious programs or beliefs into the wheel, you have a clearer understanding of why things haven't been working the way you'd like them to work.

Often we think of our life happening as if all the elements are random and out of our control. However, as we examine our underlying programs and beliefs, we find that our outer world is a reflection of what we hold to be true in our inner world.

Let's apply this to the equation of your health, using the example of stress at work. You may find that the stress you experience at work is fueled by an underlying feeling or pressure to be perfect. This feeling may then point to the underlying belief, "If I am perfect, I will be worthy of love" or "If I'm not perfect, I'm not worthy of love." Clearing up the underlying belief may actually clear up the whole stress cycle: If I don't need to be perfect and I'm okay with who I am, I feel less stress at work.

Feeling less stress at work means I can think more clearly and so I am more productive. As I feel more productive, I become proud of my accomplishments and feel better about myself. As I feel better about myself, I find I'm more motivated to eat right, which gives me more health and energy, which increases my motivation for working out, which causes me to feel more balanced and centered when I get home. Because I feel better, I have better communication with my spouse and thus a better relationship.

As you notice your underlying thoughts and feelings about yourself, you can begin to question the thoughts that aren't working for you. As you question them, you'll begin to identify many of them as being not real – they are just old ideas you chose to pick up through the journey of life.

Beliefs Operate as Self-Fulfilling Prophecies

Here's how these defining beliefs affect our daily experiences. They are responsible for many of the recurring experiences in our lives. They act like self-fulfilling prophecies.

If I have an underlying belief that I am not attractive, I may find myself feeling more self-conscious in meeting new people, which then causes me to be shy or withdrawn. Being shy causes me to avoid eye contact, which sends others the message that I am not interested in meeting them. This body language keeps me from meeting new people. From this, the mind interprets it as, "People don't want to meet me so I must not be attractive enough," which reinforces the old belief.

These underlying beliefs are responsible for the patterns of many areas of life. If I don't feel good enough, that self-fulfilling prophecy may be reflected in my career, my relationship, my family and friends, and my self-care habits.

By noticing the core beliefs that define who you think you are and changing them, you can finally take charge of the patterns running your life. As you upgrade your internal beliefs, you will create an internal sense of feeling okay, a greater sense of well-being and balance. Not only will you feel better, but also it will be easier for you to make your life work.

Especially powerful are your "I am" beliefs. You are the authority on you, and who you think you are is the most important opinion of you out there! As you feel better about yourself, you naturally make better choices that support you. The choices you make every day are reflections of these deeply held beliefs.

Who we think we are is central to how our life works. Often we define ourselves by our past – our choices and experiences. But when we've experienced something and it becomes the past, it is then only a memory. If the definitions of who we are come from the past, they are simply outdated.

Defining who we are by old memories keeps us stuck in the past. The past doesn't define who we are. The past only shapes our perspective. You are more than any feeling; you are more than any experience or even the sum of your experiences.

The past does not define us-it can only shape our perspective, and we always have choice in our perspectives.

You can dump the old ideas and the baggage that doesn't serve you. It's time to redefine yourself as your best! Don't let your life continue to be run by others' ideas and opinions, however well intentioned they might be.

Who you think you are makes all the difference. You get to decide who you are. Our lives are a reflection of who we think we are and what we think we can accomplish.

What if rather than defining yourself by the past, you used

your vision of your brightest, highest picture of yourself to define who you are? How would that change how you see yourself? How we see ourselves translates into our daily choices. If we set our mind to operate from a positive mindset and clear out the old beliefs and ideas that are no longer working, we can come to the clarity of living life on our own terms, being more at choice in what we think and feel and do.

As you rewrite the old habits and patterns, especially the beliefs at the unconscious level, you will find you have more choice in your life and feel better about yourself, and you can move forward in creating a life you love!

We are meant to live healthy, happy lives, pursuing our dreams and bringing our contributions to the world. Our body is our vehicle for living out our life purpose. You only get one body, so nourish yourself on all levels: physically, mentally, emotionally, socially and spiritually.

As you take the time for taking care of yourself, you'll begin to feel a new relationship to our body. Ideally, we want our body to naturally balance our weight and our health so we can get to living what's really important.

Grow Your Happiness

As we feel better, we do better. When we are happy and fulfilled, we reach out to others, we are kind, we are compassionate, and we are motivated! Happiness is the fuel for being our best self.

When we think about happiness, often we choose a goal that we think will bring us happiness. Then, we go through the Life Cycle of a Goal (in Chapter One) and maybe achieve some progress; but more often than not, we fall off the wagon and feel worse. Because we haven't achieved the goal, we don't deserve the reward and so we think we don't deserve to feel happy or whatever positive feeling we think the goal would bring.

Stop putting your happiness out into the land of someday, thinking "I will be happy when I have a new relationship or when I get a raise or when I have a new car or when I have a new house or . . . ." The problem with this line of thinking is that even when we achieve the new house or the new car, we might be happy for a short while, but then we find a new condition for our happiness. We set new boundaries and limitations on our happiness by defining a goal.

At any given time in life, we have both positives and negatives. We have things working for us and things seemingly working against us at the same time. Do you focus on what isn't working, or do you focus on what is working? Every day we choose where we place our focus, and what we focus on will grow.

What we focus on will grow. If you want to grow the happiness in your life, focus on happiness.

The secret is, you can access any positive feeling you want just by thinking about it. You can choose happiness now, though it might take some mental work to get there. It can be as simple as connecting with a feeling of happiness, remembering a time and place that you felt happy, or even feeling gratitude. The feelings of appreciation and gratitude are very similar to the emotion of happiness.

Happiness is a perspective, not a goal or a destination. An essential key to happiness is appreciating and loving who you are. Be kind with yourself. If you are not feeling good about yourself, it radiates into all areas of your life. If you feel positive about you, that positive energy also radiates into all areas of your life.

Happiness starts with being clear with yourself. Have compassion for yourself and your past. We are all trying to live our best. It's easy to look to the past with regret and say, if only I had chosen something else instead. Recognize that the choices you made in the past were the best choices available to you at the time with what you knew. And, as you are always learning and growing, you are now better able to make better choices.

We are all learning and growing on this planet earth. No one is expected to be perfect, just like we wouldn't expect a child to be perfect in riding a bicycle for the first time. Life is lived by learning and growing and making adjustments along the way.

Happiness is being okay with the past, loving who you are in the present, and looking forward to your future with enthusiasm.

If you criticize yourself, if you don't feel good about who you are, look for negative programs such as the "I am" beliefs you have picked up – and change them. Examine your expectations. Are they realistic? Are your underlying beliefs and programs supporting you in living a happy and fulfilled life?

Love and accept yourself in the present moment. You can revisit the exercise for appreciation, love and awe in chapter one. Accepting yourself in the present moment is to surrender to whatever your situation is at the moment. Rather than resisting it, or struggling with what you don't like about your situation, simply accept it.

Ask yourself, "what is there to appreciate about this situation?"

If you are single, this time of transition is a great time to reflect on what is really important to you in your life. When you focus on what there is to appreciate in your life rather than struggling with what you don't have, you tune your brain to appreciation and happiness.

No matter where you are - there you are. No matter where you are in life, it's just a starting point, or a stepping stone on the path to what's next for you. Resist the temptation to compare your situation with others. Appreciating what others have can be a cue for you to recognize what you want, but don't make yourself less than someone else because of what you have or don't have.

Look forward to your future with enthusiasm.

What does the future look like to you? When you picture stepping out into the future, how does your brain represent that in images, pictures, sounds and feelings?

Our ability to imagine is the cornerstone of creation. If you can imagine something, you can then set about creating it. Everything in our lives now is the result of someone's imagination. What do you imagine for yourself in your future?

If the future you picture is dull or gloomy, what can you add to the picture that would make it come alive and be vibrant and compelling for you?

When I was first learning NLP, we did an exercise of envisioning our future. When I thought about the future, it looked dark and gloomy to me, as if there was no path forward. My mind was operating from a fear of the future, so I had a hard time picturing the future in my mind.

But changing this is simple. Try this exercise in NLP style.

Imagine seeing an image of your best future. Imagine one year from now, what would you like to see in your life? What is in that picture? What people do you see there, what activities, what environments? What would you be saying to yourself in that positive future? What would you be feeling in that positive future?

And now, you can add some things to enhance it. What if you added more light to the visual picture, how does that affect the future? What if you added flowers - how does that change it? Now add some sounds, add laughter in the background, how does that enhance it? Maybe add more color or texture, what if you added softness to it, or silken smooth texture?

And, I always like to add a pinch of pixie dust for good measure! How does that change how you feel about the future?

If, when you think of the future, you are not inspired and excited, it is simply telling you to make a change. Sometimes the best change we can make is not action, but perception.

If you don't like your reality - change your perception!

We are always at choice. At any one time, we have a myriad of options available to us. We first choose our perspective, and then we make our lives match that which we think is true.

If you are not happy in your life, start noticing – what perspectives and what thoughts are keeping you stuck? Look specifically for any negative beliefs, such as, I don't deserve it, I'm not good enough, or I can't because…. Once you change these underlying beliefs it will give you great momentum in really moving forward toward anything you want in life.

It's not so much our situation, but the stories we use to describe it that become our mental roadblocks. If you don't like the situation, change your story about it.

Keep A Feel Good Journal

One way to train your brain to be more positive is to give your attention to what you want your brain to focus on. As you remind yourself to think positive thoughts, you'll be feeling more positive feelings, you'll be inspired and motivated to take positive actions which then help you think better thoughts and feel better feelings.

It creates an upward spiral for thinking better, feeling better and then taking positive action. Keep a small notebook with you and take the time to review it daily. It's a great way to start off your day or review it a few times throughout the day to keep your positive mindset.

Memories Inspire Happiness

Keep pages in your journal for a list of all the things, people, places, and memories that inspire a feeling of happiness. As you review the list, you'll notice the feeling of these happy memories returning.

Exercise Your Gratitude

Gratitude and happiness are like muscles: the more you use exercise them, the stronger they become.

Keep a list of the things for which you are grateful. Gratitude and happiness are very closely related. Being grateful for what's working in your life can bring you closer to happiness. Start your gratitude pages by finding at least 10 things to be grateful for and keep adding them to your list.

What do you Appreciate

Keep pages in your journal for what you appreciate. You can make a section specifically for what you appreciate about you: what are your gifts and talents and what do you do well? As we appreciate ourselves, we feel more expansive in who we are and we are more likely to be motivated, give our best and reach out to others.

Keep a page on what you appreciate about your life. What is working for you in your life? What can you appreciate? It can be as simple as appreciating your bed, your home or the people in your life. If you are feeling frustrated with your partner, listing out the positive qualities and characteristics will help you focus on the positives and may even shift your frustrations, allowing you to enjoy your relationship even more.

When we come from a mindset of appreciation, we tune our brain into the positives, we carry positive energy and that mindset brings out the best in those around us. From this positive mindset, we notice more of what's working in our lives and we are better able to find the positive solutions to the problems we may experience.

Too often we get caught up in the daily grind mindset and we miss the many miracles that surround us. By bringing your attention to appreciate the mundane things in life, you shift your focus to seeing the many miracles around you every day.

Do What You Love

In *Flow*, Hungarian psychologist Csíkszentmihályi Mihalyi describes happiness as a state of flow, when we are engrossed in a task or endeavor for its own sake and we experience a sense of timelessness. Athletes often refer to this state as being in the zone. In what activities do you experience flow and timelessness?

Make a list of activities that nourish you and inspire happiness. What are the activities, the people, the places, and the events that inspire a feeling of happiness for you? Set aside time in your schedule to do the activities you love.

Spend more time doing the things that you truly love and enjoy. If you gave yourself time during your week for you, what would that look like?

To connect with happiness and well being, you don't have to take hours out of your week, though that would be a great idea too. It can be as simple as taking 5 minutes to review your journal and connect with the positive thoughts that will bring you the positive feelings.

Our Imagination Speaks to Our Unconscious

As we use our imagination for what we'd like to see in our lives, it speaks to our unconscious mind and in a sense, paves the way for us to achieve that reality.

As we imagine our positive future, it tunes our brain into that reality. Our brain then pays attention to the very things that will help us move forward.

Imagine seeing your positive healthy future. Engage the visual, auditory and kinesthetic cues for engaging your brain and tuning into that reality.

What will you be seeing?

What will you be saying to yourself or hearing?

What will you be feeling?

What more do you see for yourself as you are making healthier and healthier choices day by day?

And now, bring that future back to you now in the present moment, and as you do, your unconscious mind can lay out that roadmap for staying connected with this positive vision of you. As we picture a positive, vibrant future, we find a wellspring of motivation. Fuel your motivation by imagining your best life.

The Magic of Asking Questions

Any time we ask a question, our mind has to go find the answer. If you ask the right kinds of questions, your mind will respond with positive and helpful information and positive feelings. Here are some positive questions you can begin asking yourself. As you read these questions, notice how you feel in response. Give a pause after reading each question and notice what responses come to mind.

What is my health potential?

What is possible for me?

How would it be to be my ideal healthy weight?

Who am I becoming as the lighter, freer self?

As you can see, these questions inspire the positive feelings of embodying your ideal healthy weight. As you connect with these positive feelings, it tunes your brain into that reality. These positive feelings are also the fuel of motivation that keeps us going.

Cultivate Aliveness with Childlike Curiosity

Have you seen the light and wonder in a child's eyes when they are experiencing something new? One time I was visiting my nieces and nephews and I heard shrieking from the garden, so I went out to see what all the ruckus was about. My niece, Jerusha, 7 years old and nephew, Tor, who was 5, were taking turns holding an earthworm and as it wiggled in their hands, they were shrieking with excitement. As I looked down at the earthworm, I almost said, "It's just an earthworm," but I bit my tongue. As I saw their delight and intensity, I wondered, what would it be like to see the worm through their eyes?

As I thought of that, I saw a whole new dimension for the earthworm, the pulsating veins on its sides changing colors. I asked if I could hold the worm, and Jerusha plopped it into my hand. As she did, the worm twisted and wiggled, and I could feel its wetness and coldness squirming against my hand. I focused on the sensation of it, on the feel of its squirming and the excitement that this little pink line of flesh that was alive wiggling in the palm of my hand.

For a few magical moments, the three of us were enthralled with the squirmy pink worm. If I had said, "It's just an earthworm" I would have killed the moment, and I would have missed experiencing the magic with them.

As adults it seems that we let the newness and magic of life fade. But all we need to bring back that wonder of life is to be curious.

How much in life do we take for granted because it is familiar? Even if you've seen it a hundred times, what is new about this time?

How much in our lives have we stopped exploring or being open to new moments or new experiences because we think we know something? What if you were to view the people in your life with curiosity, who are they now in this moment? And how might that change your experience with them?

What aliveness can you bring to your life now by just being curious? What magic can you see in the small moments of life?

Life Enjoyment

I wonder what there is for me to enjoy today? What a great question with which to start your day.

Thinking of all the small miracles, the sensations, the gifts, the inventions, the products, the tools, the comforts, the pleasures, the conveniences, the technology, the nature, the animals, the people...there is so much to enjoy!

When we ask the question, "What is there for me to enjoy?" the mind goes to find the answer. As you ask the question, you are tuning your brain into life enjoyment.

What do you want to experience today? What positive feelings do you want your brain to notice for you?

Happiness As a Skill

I tend to think of happiness as a skill, something we can exercise and practice. By using awareness and changing your mental and emotional habits and beliefs, you can experience greater well being and expand the happiness in all areas of your life.

The interesting thing about the brain is that the brain's ability to access our memories depends on our current emotional state. So, if you are thinking positively and feeling happy, you'll have a greater ability to remember your happy memories. If you are sad and depressed, your mind accesses the memories that mirror that emotional state.

So, as you practice your happiness and your positive state of mind, you are also tuning your brain into more positive thinking. Besides, being positive is just more fun and it feels better.

If you struggle with difficult emotions, I suggest you review the material in Chapter Four that will help you process those emotions so that you can be more at choice in what you are feeling. As you take the time to work through your emotions, you'll begin to feel clearer with less emotional interference throughout your day.

Who are you as the Ideal Healthy Self

Don't put off your happiness until you've attained your goal weight. Love and appreciate who you are now, and you'll enjoy the journey of getting there even more. You will be with yourself for the entire journey of life, so you might as well appreciate your own company.

It's time to let go of old definitions of ourselves, of old baggage that holds us back, and begin to see ourselves how we would like to be. Let's define ourselves by our highest potential rather than by outdated memories. Even though you may see a difference between where you are now and where you would like to be, you can appreciate who you are now and you'll enjoy the journey of getting there so much more.

As you define yourself by your potential and your possibilities rather than by old definitions of the past, you can truly embrace life and step into your potential.

In fact, we are learning and growing every day. We are making new choices every day, and we are even choosing who we are every day. We are always choosing. If something isn't working for you in your life, it's time to make a new choice. Sometimes the most powerful choice you can make is a new perspective.

Who would you like to be? Write some I am statements about who you are becoming as your highest and best vision of you. What would you like to embrace in your life?

I am healthy and active.

I love my body.

It feels good to be me.

I can slim down to my ideal healthy weight.

Working with your Unconscious Mind

Think of your unconscious mind as a highly compact super-computer able to process large amounts of information very quickly. The unconscious mind holds the grand archives of all your past history, and it is responsible for taking in much more information than you can consciously process. Have you ever met someone and you had a feeling about that person, but couldn't place the reason as to why you felt that way about them? This is your unconscious mind at work, it sums up all the information, the subtle cues of body language, the voice inflections, the minor movements, and compares the person to people you've met in the past that are similar - and then you get a feeling about that person.

The unconscious mind is also responsible for running automatic programs of the body and body processes. Your body itself has an inherent wisdom about what nutrients you are absorbing and what nutrients your body needs at any given time. Your unconscious mind can process that information instantaneously.

In our western culture, there is a rift between the conscious mind and the subconscious mind. We are not used to checking in with our deeper awareness. But we can access the greater wisdom of the unconscious mind and body very quickly simply by asking.

The unconscious mind tends to like pictures, images, symbols, metaphors, more than words, but everyone experiences responses from the unconscious in different ways. Some people get more visual responses, some people get more auditory or sound responses, and some people get more feeling or sensing responses. Just pay attention to how you receive the information.

Intuitive Eating

You can ask your unconscious mind directly, "I ask my unconscious mind to let me know what foods will help me reach my ideal weight even more quickly."

After asking this question, imagine a movie screen in your mind's eye, and ask your unconscious mind to project onto that movie screen the foods that will help you speed your healthy body results.

You can also do this exercise while shopping, and notice what foods seem to stand out for you and what foods you are drawn to.

Sometimes with this exercise, you might get information that the foods your unconscious mind is picturing are not the healthy foods that you might expect. When these come up, ask the question, "What do I really want?" and notice what response you get. It will probably be a feeling.

Give yourself the positive feeling and then notice if the craving subsides. If the craving doesn't subside, it may be that you only need a small amount of that food.

One story comes from Sally, she had taken my course, and she found exercise that she really enjoyed, Zumba. But, she also found that after Zumba, she would just crave potato chips. When she asked the question, "What do I really want?" she just kept getting pictures of potato chips. So, she opted for a handful and as she was eating them, the salt just tasted amazing to her.

Her body was craving the salt to replace the electrolytes she had lost through the intense physical activity. She took a small handful of salt and after a couple licks of it, felt satisfied and no longer wanted the potato chips.

Intuitive Eating - Adopting Curiosity

Body chemistry is different for everyone. What your body needs may not be the same as the next person. There are principles of healthy eating and nutrition, but as you pay attention to what your body wants, you'll begin to be aware of the foods that your body needs to rebalance itself.

I used to have a lot of sugar cravings. My mom was a great cook and we always had desserts after dinner. This became a habit that overrode the "I'm full" signal. I didn't think I was finished eating until after I had eaten dessert.

Now, I find myself actually craving brussel sprouts, beet greens, and green smoothies. There is something so fulfilling and satisfying in really enjoying the depth of flavors in healthy foods that your body wants.

I still enjoy treats and desserts, but not in the way that I used to. I allow myself to really dive into the flavors, textures and sensations of the first few bites. I love soaking up the feeling of it. And then, after a couple of bites, I notice I'm done. It's easy to put it down and walk away.

Intuitive eating is paying attention to your body, the foods it wants, and recognizing the difference between cravings and habits versus what your body actually wants.

Mindfulness eating is about being aware of your body while you are eating. Be totally present with the flavors, the textures, diving into the awareness of the foods that you are eating. As you do, you will even notice subtleties of the nutrients that your body wants and needs to maintain your health and energy.

I love taking some quiet time with my meals, and just focusing on the flavors, sometimes it's even euphoric to really dive into the tastes, the flavors, and really appreciate the textures.

How many meals have you had where you plow through and get to the end of the meal only to notice that you hardly tasted it?

When we do other things while we are eating, we rob our attention of food. If you eat while watching TV, your attention isn't on the food. If you eat on the run, go through fast food, eat in the car, you are not really enjoying your food.

In the CD, Curb Your Cravings, we ask your unconscious mind to rewire from cravings to preferring healthy foods and healthy choices. This also has some mental exercises to help you naturally reach for those foods that are good for your body.

Explore More Fruits and Vegetables With Curiosity

Part of the reason that we don't crave things that are good for us is that we are limited in what foods our body is used to, especially if we've been emotionally driven by our food choices in the past.

When you go to the produce aisle of the grocery store, what foods do you usually put in your cart? Usually we put the same 20 or so items into the cart every time, we get into routines in our food choices. The next time you are in the grocery store, take a look around and notice what fruits or vegetables you haven't tried or the produce that is unfamiliar to you and try some new things.

Sometimes we've decided we don't like certain foods, but our tastes can change over time. I hated onions as a kid and my mom put them in everything, I had to constantly pick them out of my dinners. Now, as an adult, I love onions and I could eat them with every meal.

If you have certain fruits or vegetables that you don't like, make an experiment to see if you still don't like them as an adult or see if your tastes have changed.

If you adopt a mindset of curiosity, simply ask your mind and your body: how does this taste to me, or what does my body like about this? You'll get an even deeper sense of satisfaction. Or, you may find you simply don't like that food or flavor.

I used to be a pasta lover. Italian food and pasta was one of my favorite things. As I began to ask my body what it liked, pasta took on a sense of being white, pasty, and blah. It didn't have the same appeal to me that it had before. I still eat pasta from time to time, but not in the frequency that I used to.

As you care for yourself on all levels, your body will be clearer with you about what foods and nutrients you need to feel your best.

Ending the Struggle with your Body

In the old paradigm of weight loss, we map out a plan of what we will do, what we will eat, and then we think we need more discipline to make ourselves stay on track.

In the old paradigm of weight loss, we are at war with our bodies. We struggle against ourselves, our cravings, the lack of motivation, and we beat ourselves up for not staying on track with a program. We wonder why we can't just make ourselves do it.

Instead of getting caught up in the guilt and self criticism, we can look at our habits and behaviors with the light of awareness and ask, "what is this telling me?" Your 'failures' are simply useful information pointing to something that isn't working for you.

If you are experiencing self sabotage or not following through, it simply means that some part of you wants attention.

Rather than fight and struggle against our cravings, we can ask that part of us, "what do I really want?"

Now, with the tools of self awareness, you can identify what you want and nourish yourself on all levels, physically, mentally, emotionally, and spiritually.

What if your cravings were simply messengers of what you want more of in your life? What if your cravings were telling you about how to live a more fulfilling and balanced life?

Rather than struggling against cravings, you can now recognize your messages, and move forward with positive awareness. If cravings for you are about life happiness, then your system is asking for more focus on life happiness.

Make time for yourself. Create space in your schedule to connect with life happiness. Maybe one hour on the weekend to do things that make you happy. Reviewing your Feel Good Journal daily will help keep your mindset in the positive.

Befriend Your Body

In the old model of weight loss, we are at war with our bodies. We have to force it into submission with exhaustive hours at the gym. We deprive it and deny it the foods that it craves, like sweets and fats and carbohydrates. But lasting weight loss doesn't have to be such a struggle. In fact, lasting weight loss success requires building a relationship with your body that is positive.

It's time to end the war with your body. Your body is a vehicle for you to enjoy life, to live your life purpose and bring your contribution to the world. Your body is actually working for you. What if your cravings were just messengers of what you want out of life?

When we gain weight, we tend to criticize and berate ourselves. We judge ourselves for the extra weight. We judge others for the extra weight. We may even think we have less worth or value in who we are if we weigh more than we'd like.

Your body will be with you your whole life. Start to make friends with it. Appreciate it for what it does for you everyday. It works for you automatically every day, regulating subtle changes such as pH balance, heart rate, respirations, blood pressure, body temperature, and it does all of this automatically.

Your body has inherent wisdom. Your systems all communicate with each other, and work together to keep you in balance and keep your system in equilibrium. Recognize and appreciate your body for what it is doing for you. This will start to build a positive relationship with your body. How do you feel when you are appreciated? You feel good, expansive and more willing to express yourself.

When you are criticized and belittled, how do you feel then? You feel small, you hold yourself back, and feel withdrawn. As you focus on appreciating your body, its inherent wisdom engages with you at the unconscious level and comes into alignment with our conscious goals.

Create a Relationship with Your Body

If you want your body's wisdom to work for you, you need to let it know that you are on its side. Your body already knows how to regulate and heal itself, and as you look through your history and find many examples of how it has done this for you automatically.

Your body has continued to create balance day by day through all its processes.

Give your body the right mental environment that allows it to release the excess weight for you. Praise your body for all that it's doing well now. In fact, read the following out loud to yourself:

Thank you body for automatically regulating my heart rate.

Thank you body for automatically regulating my blood pressure.

Thank you body for automatically regulating my oxygen levels.

Thank you body for automatically taking oxygen to every little cell.

Thank you body for automatically digesting my food and absorbing nutrients.

Thank you body for automatically taking nutrients to every cell of my body.

Thank you body for automatically creating new cells to replace the old ones.

Thank you body for automatically regulating my pH levels.

Thank you body for automatically flushing out what I don't need.

How does your body feel to be acknowledged and appreciated?

You are amazing aren't you? Now, notice how you feel about your body. Isn't your body fantastic?

Rather than pushing yourself into intense physical activity, you might ask your body what it wants to do for exercise, what does it enjoy?

I connect with different exercises depending on the mood I'm in. Somedays, I really enjoy a 10 or 20 minute meditative walk. Other days, I love the thrill of all out sprinting or running.

Yoga is great exercise for developing the mental connection to your body. There are many styles and disciplines of yoga. I took a Kripalu yoga class in college, and I remember that's where I really connected with the mind and body connection, I really saw my body as a living entity rather than a hunk of flesh to carry around with me.

In Kripalu yoga, you initially go through certain poses and postures, but then you simply open up the space and time to move how your body wants to move. Maybe it goes into postures and flows, or maybe you find yourself holding a new pose or stretch. It really engages a question and answer between you and your body. It's like a moving meditation, flowing with the movement of the body. I often dip into timelessness with the movement, which is nourishing not only for the body, but also for the mind and spirit as well.

Give yourself some variety in your workouts and movements and try some new classes to explore with curiosity. What kinds of exercise and movements do you enjoy? Finding the right exercise for you can be as simple as asking your body, what would it like to do today?

What exercises and activities actually give you joy? I love dancing, moving with the rhythm of the music.

Nourish Yourself on All Levels

Make yourself a priority. So many of us have picked up the idea or the message that it's better to take care of others first.

When we are depleted of energy, when we are doing things we don't want to do, or feel obligated to do, we have less energy to share with others. When we feel resentful about what we are doing, we are snippy, ornery, and short with others.

When we feel good about who we are, we feel energized. When we take care of ourselves and fill our energy reserves, we then naturally reach out to others.

What activities nourish and support you?

Make time for yourself.

Congratulations on making your way through this book. I hope you've found some helpful tools that you've started applying to reach the lighter, happier you.

Remember, achieving and maintaining your ideal weight is a journey, but it doesn't have to be a struggle. It's the small steps you take every day that really add up. Appreciate all the steps you've already taken that are positive and that are moving you in a better direction day by day. Every positive choice and action is one step closer to that healthier, happier you.

Review of the Shortcuts

Your brain has habits wired in by the neuronal pathways of the neurons in your brain.

Repetition helps your brain create new habits.

Your cravings are messengers for what you want more of in life.

Emotions are messengers giving you useful information.

Work through the layers of emotions to transform the negative feelings and get to the positive ones.

Self sabotage points to unconscious programs that aren't working for you.

Examine your beliefs about what it means to be healthy, about your body.

Your "I am" beliefs are core to how your life operates.

Expand your sense of life fulfillment using the Life Balance Wheel.

Identify where your weight is asking you to expand your fulfillment and well being.

Make time to connect with positive feelings through a mindset journal.

Grow your happiness, your appreciation, your well being.

Make time for yourself.

Appendix

Exercises and NLP Tools

Other Considerations

The weight equation can be complicated. Foundational to your success is your mindset, your habits, meanings, and even unconscious programs for which I've discussed effective tools in this book. If you are not getting the results you want, here's some other things to consider for moving forward. More information about each of these areas can be found on the website: www.ALigterYouSystem.com

Nutrition: You simply cannot have a real conversation about your health without talking about the quality of the foods you are choosing. It's like wanting peak performance from your car, but only giving it bad gas. There are certain things our body needs to perform optimally. Because you live in a body, and it's the only one you have for your entire life, take time to learn about what your body needs for optimal health. Take responsibility to be informed; don't wait until you are sick or have a health crisis. Learn about your body and what it needs. Visit my website for the nutrition guide.

Slow Metabolism: Calorie-restrictive diets can actually lower your metabolism 10-15 percent. If your body temperature runs on the cold side, if you feel tired and sluggish, a slow metabolism could be a factor. By eating low-glycemic foods and quality whole foods, you can correct a slow metabolism and get your body back into the fat-burning zone. Hormonal imbalances may also contribute to a slow metabolism. Have your hormone levels checked by a qualified health care professional.

Food Allergies and Sensitivities: You can have food sensitivities without having a full-blown allergy. These sensitivities and allergies can cause a wide range of symptoms as well as cause your body to retain extra water weight and fat. Food allergies and sensitivities are on the rise, and I think we will continue to see an increase. Because the symptoms can be subtle, you could be living for years with a food sensitivity and not know it. Sensitivities may not show up on blood allergy tests, but by paying attention to what you are eating and how you feel, you can identify the foods that don't work well for you.

Stress: When we are stressed, our body releases hormones, namely cortisol and adrenaline. If these hormone levels remain high over time, cortisol can actually cause us to gain weight and store extra fat. To help your body release fat, you will need to address your stress levels. Train Your Brain for Stress Relief CD can help set up new patterns in your brain around stress so that you experience greater calm and well being in your life.

Toxins: Accumulations of toxins over time can interfere with the body's ability to normalize weight. The body may store toxins in fat and tissues. You may find a good detoxification system useful in helping your body kick-start its metabolism and release the fat. However, recognize that a detox system is not a substitution for healthy eating. What you eat is the foundation to your health, your body's balance and your energy.

Tools and Resources

Visit the website www.ALighterYouSystem.com for more information about the following products, tools, and resources.

The Online A Lighter You! Membership program includes audios, live question and answer calls, recorded calls and tele-classes, articles, access to hypnosis archives and more to help you transform the negative patterns and stay motivated.

Tele-classes run periodically, look online for the next starting dates.

The six-part audio set *A Lighter You! Mind Body Weight Loss Audio Course* helps chronic dieters change the old habits in what you think, feel, and do. Train your brain to create new habits and you'll find making healthy choices easier and easier. With this audio course, you can even train your brain while you sleep! Here's the titles and descriptions of the six CDs in the set:

Step Into Your Healthy You helps gives your unconscious mind the roadmap to your lighter, freer self so you can slim down naturally.

Curb Your Cravings gives your mind a new focus for choosing foods, plus mental strategies to prefer healthy foods and curb your cravings.

Enlighten Your Body Image helps you release negative labels and self criticisms that have weighed you down and held you back. This CD also helps you internalize a sense of comfort and well being, thus curbing the compulsion for comfort eating.

Motivation for Fitness helps you maintain a positive focus with exercise so that you look forward to a great workout.

Boost Your Metabolism gives your mind and body a positive focus for increasing your energy, harmonizing your body systems and boosting your metabolism.

Release Your Reasons gives your unconscious mind a gentle and effective way to release the negative ideas and beliefs you have picked up about weight, health and your body.

In my guide, *A Lighter You! The Health Coach's Guide to Nutrition in Action: How to Eat Your Way to a Slimmer You*, you'll find step-by-step guidelines for nutrition information, how to eat for health and energy, and how to slim your body through food for lasting weight loss success.

Would you like to be A Lighter You Coach? See the website for the facilitator training schedule.

If you feel stuck, you'll find working with a qualified Master NLP practitioner very helpful. Find one in your area. I also work with clients by phone all across the United States. See the website for details on booking a starter session.

What's Next

This is only the beginning! You can apply the same tools to any area of your life in which you want to make a change. We have habits in our relationships, our jobs or careers, how we handle money or stress, health, and more. Underneath these habits we have thought patterns and feeling patterns that drive the behaviors. Underneath these we even have unconscious programs and beliefs and even "I am" beliefs about who we are that direct how we operate in the world.

What more do you want for yourself?

• Greater Life Purpose

• Increased Health or Illness Recovery

• Increased Work & Career Fulfillment

• Expansion in Money & Finances

• Greater Focus & Motivation

Are you ready to live your life's purpose with more clarity, insight, and passion? You really can have the life you want! By making changes in how you operate, by changing your mental and emotional habits, your meanings and beliefs and the definitions of you, you can profoundly change your experience and create a life that you love.

I love working on the deeper level of changing beliefs and old programs, because as we adjust these areas, we increase the ability for true happiness and expand our potential. As we help the brain learn new habits and patterns, it can be working for us, setting us up for success!

With the right tools and the right support, you can have the life, the health, the body, the career, the wealth, and life fulfillment you desire. It's time to believe in your best life and train your brain to get you there!

Here's to your Health, Happiness, and Success!

Holly Stokes, The Brain Trainer

NLP References

Andreas, Connirae and Tamara Andreas. *Core Transformation: Reaching the Wellspring Within.* 1994. Real People Press, Moab, UT.

Andreas, Steve and Charles Faulkner. *NLP The New Technology of Achievement.* 1994. NLP Comprehensive. New York, NY

Dilts, Robert; Tim Halbom and Suzi Smith. *Beliefs: Pathways to Health and Well-being.* 1990, Metamorphous Press, Portland, OR.

Dilts, Robert. *From Coach to Awakener.* 2003. Metapublications, Capitola, CA.

Hall, L. Michael. *Secrets of Personal Mastery.* 1997. Wales, UK: Crown house Publications.

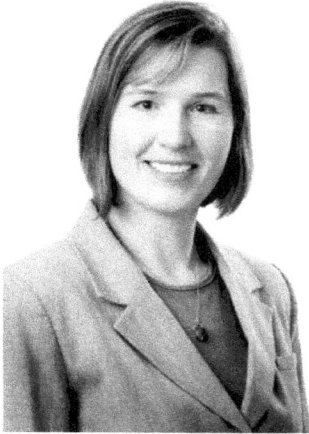

About the Author

Holly Stokes, aka The Brain Trainer, is a Master Neuro-Linguistic Programming (NLP) health coach and certified hypnotherapist. She began working in the field of personal development in 1994, teaching at-risk youth communication skills, motivation, and leadership.

Her work in this area led her to finish her degree in psychology at Portland State University in Portland, Oregon. While finishing her psychology coursework, she found the NLP coaching and hypnotherapy tools. She was amazed at how quickly these tools helped clients change old habits, negative thinking and replace negative patterns and beliefs. She began working as The Brain Trainer in 2005.

As a speaker she inspires audiences in motivation, work-life balance, changing habits, health and wellness, and creating the mindset for success. She lives in the Salt Lake City Utah and works with clients all across the United States by phone.

Holly is passionate about empowering clients to overcome their obstacles, change the old patterns, and start living their best life now.

Services Offered:

Private Sessions

Group Coaching and Online Programs

Motivational Speaker

Holly continues to develop products to help clients achieve their potential in life happiness, health, wealth, and business.

Discover more and follow her blog at:
http://www.BrainTrainerCoach.com

Weight Loss Website: www.ALighterYouSystem.com

Email Holly at: Holly@BrainTrainerCoach.com

Follow Holly on Twitter: www.twitter.com/hollystokes

Fan Page on Facebook:
http://www.facebook.com/TheBrainTrainerLLC

A Lighter You! Train Your Brain to Slim Your Body